DUE

Aug 18 1995

Evaluation of Pregnancy Prevention Programs in the School Context

Evaluation of Pregnancy Prevention Programs in the School Context

Laurie Schwab Zabin
The Johns Hopkins School of Hygiene and Public Health

Marilyn B. Hirsch
The Johns Hopkins School of Medicine

Lexington Books
D.C. Heath and Company/Lexington, Massachusetts/Toronto

Library of Congress Cataloging-in-Publication Data

Zabin, Laurie Schwab.
  School-based pregnancy prevention programs.

  Includes index.
  1. Johns Hopkins Adolescent Pregnancy Prevention Program.   2. Pregnancy, Adolescent—
Maryland—Baltimore.
3. Birth control—Maryland—Baltimore.   4. Sex instruction for youth—Maryland—
Baltimore.   5. Evaluation research (Social action programs)—Maryland—
Baltimore.   I. Hirsch, Marilyn B.   II. Title. [DNLM: 1. Evaluation Studies.
2. Pregnancy in Adolescence.   3. School Health Services—United States.   4. Sex
Education—United States.
WS 462 Z12s]
LB3432.Z33   1987   362.8′392′088055   86–46359
ISBN 0–669–15844–5 (alk. paper)

Published simultaneously in Canada
Printed in the United States of America
International Standard Book Number: 0–669–15844–5
Library of Congress Catalog Card Number: 86–46359

The paper used in this publication meets the minimum requirements of American National
Standard for Information Sciences—Permanence of Paper for Printed Library Materials, ANSI
Z39.48–1984. ⊗™

88 89 90 91 8 7 6 5 4 3 2 1

Contents

Preface

The program on which the methods presented here were honed was the work of many. Conceived by Janet B. Hardy, M.D.C.M., and directed by Rosalie Streett, M.S., it reflected their commitment of many years to adolescent services, their warmth of caring, their experience, their judgement, and their skill. The team they assembled included for the duration of the project Ellen Hoffman Goldwasser, M.S.W., Marcia Chapman Gratton, C.N.M., and Bernadette Butler, Registrar; at one time period or another, Mary Lou Curran, P.N.P., Nancy Mackenzie, P.N.P., Chris Fitzgerald, M.S.W., and Esther Vines, M.S.W., were a part of the dedicated staff. Theodore M. King, M.D., Ph.D., served as Clinician; as Chairman of the Department of Gynecology and Obstetrics, he has long supported the notion that the social science of reproduction is an important component of that medical discipline. Without the understanding of the program staff, not only of the students but of the demanding evaluation team, this experiment could not have resulted in the research model we present in this book. To them, and to those like them throughout the country who serve our young people with their hearts and with their minds, who are brave enough to address tough problems and tough enough to ask for an appraisal of what they do, this book is dedicated.

The Baltimore City School System, and especially Dr. John L. Crew who was its superintendent when this innovative program began, deserve commendation. Our warm thanks go to the principals of our four schools as well; they included Drs. Elzee Gladden, Leon Coleman, Franklin Thomas, and Donald Knox, and for a short time at the outset, Julia Woodland. The faculty of those schools also contributed, but above all our gratitude is to the students who responded so honestly and conscientiously to our "nosy" questionnaires.

The research team, too, deserves our thanks, especially Edward A. Smith, Dr. P.H., who was a colleague for much of the study period and contributed the first chapter, Mark Emerson who served as programmer, and Samuel D. Clark, Jr., Sc.M., who was with us at the beginning of the project. Susannah

Sagan, Carolyn Gehret, Andrea Chapman, and Morna Oruch worked on the data, and secretaries Nelva Hitt, Carolyn Jones, and Marsha Solomon on the hundreds of questionnaires, tables, and papers that were generated. All contributed to the endeavor. The manuscript was prepared by Beverly Siegel. Young Kim was very helpful in sorting out the statistical techniques employed in the evaluation, as was Sol Su in the programming.

Discussions with our many colleagues have helped refine the text; Claire Brindis and Douglas Kirby have shared their experiences in the schools with us; Rosalie Streett, Judith Jones, and Carolyn Anderman read the manuscript. Countless others have discussed their work and given us the feeling that our experiences were not so unique that they could not be of help to others in the field.

The techniques presented here are exhaustive and demanding. They do not need to be replicated in full to be useful; we hope they suggest a direction evaluation can go, even to those who are embarked on a different course. They are put on paper in an attempt to respond to a deluge of requests for help, too numerous to answer on an individual basis in the depth they deserve. Our questionnaires are offered to others with the hope that they may bring some standardization to the field, and with the personal hope that we will hear reports from those who utilize them elsewhere.

Our thanks must be offered to those who funded this experimental program, and gave us the time to develop a methodology that could hold up even under the scrutiny of those political opponents who seek to discredit the kinds of adolescent services that were provided. The Ford Foundation, especially, has given us this support and this freedom. The service program itself was funded by the Educational Foundation of America, which conceived the project as a service and research program from the start. The Hewlett Foundation was the first private funding source to see the potential of this evaluation. The W.T. Grant Foundation has been generous in its support of the extensive data collection and management necessary to carry out the cost effectiveness evaluation. At one time or another, the Charles Stewart Mott Foundation and the Jessie Smith Noyes Foundation have contributed as well. To each of them, and to the individuals with whom we worked within those foundations, we are deeply grateful for their support and for their trust.

Last, but not least, we thank our husbands, the late James Barton Zabin and Gary Gordon, for their love, support, and encouragement during the period that the research presented here took place.

Introduction

Since the 1960s, it has become increasingly clear that adolescent pregnancy and childbearing are major problems in the United States, out of all proportion to their significance in other countries in the Western World. During the last two decades, a considerable body of literature on the subject has developed, much of it based on sound research. The original emphases were on the epidemiology of adolescent sexuality and conception—how much, among whom—and the social, economic, and medical consequences of early childbearing. As interest has grown in many problem behaviors clustered in the teen years, associations between these problems have increasingly been the focus of research, and have given social observers the sense that, whatever the appropriate interventions may be, they need to deal with a larger objective than the prevention of premature conception alone. The time has come when there is a demand for action. Whether we have all the necessary information on which to base comprehensive programs no longer seems to be the primary issue; there is a general recognition that preventive measures need to be taken, and that we know enough to begin. The next generation of research will almost certainly be evaluative research, assessing the ability of such programs to bring about the desired change.

There has been a growing recognition that the general health needs of adolescents are often unmet; this is an age group in which, if it is received at all, medical care tends to be of a crisis nature. Awareness of the health needs of the young has coincided with interest in a more comprehensive approach to the problem of adolescent pregnancy. Simultaneously, there has been the recognition that, whatever approaches are used, initiatives need to reach the majority of, if not all, American youth—and need to reach them before problem behaviors endanger their education, their health, and, indeed, their futures. Together, these areas of understanding have led to a focus on initiatives within the school setting or closely allied with it, since the school is the only institution in regular contact with a sizeable proportion of the teenage population. Whether programs involve education or services, or some combination of the two, the school link for interventions to prevent adolescent pregnancy appears to be an important one, and, whatever difficulties there may be in the way, the concept is no doubt with us for the foreseeable future. Now there is the need to test it.

This demand for intervention, this sense of immediacy, should not imply that any unsubstantiated program will do. Useful programs tend to be expensive, and neither the funding for services nor the investment of time and money required for serious evaluation can, in the present climate, be committed without a reasonable expectation of success. However, the inclination of funders and planners to try new social experiments without much more delay is based in some degree on the fact that most of the initiatives proposed to prevent or at least to reduce the level of early childbearing are perceived as having considerable value in their own right. These initiatives, not limited in their areas of intervention to the field of reproductive health, cover adolescent services sadly in need of societal attention whether or not they have a significant impact on the adolescent pregnancy rate. What are these initiatives? Upgrading the learning experience, improving health services, broadening job opportunities, discouraging premature termination of schooling, raising educational aspiration, widening horizons for the future, involving communities in the social planning process, promoting parent-child communication, helping young people to adopt responsible preventive behaviors—all of these have been proposed as initiatives to discourage early sexual onset and premature childbearing. All have enough merit, in and of themselves, to deserve a trial. But that trial will be useful to the field only in proportion to the solid, rigorous evaluation to which it is subjected, and that implies evaluation built in as an important component from the start.

The field of adolescent services is ready to move into the generation of evaluative research, and social scientists with a serious interest in pregnancy prevention must prepare to move with it. Where will that lead? Since it has become increasingly clear that many of these initiatives can best be undertaken from a school-base, it will probably lead into the middle, junior, and senior high schools of the nation. Assessment of initiatives in diverse areas will therefore share many of the problems peculiar to that institutional setting, problems which it will be the purpose of this book to address.

The Role of Evaluation

Evaluation can serve many purposes, not the least of which is the formation of public policy. There are countless creative programs in all areas of social, education, and health service that never have the impact they might because their effects have never been put to the test of rigorous assessment. Replication often depends on proven success.

Evaluation can also serve as an administrative tool to upgrade and improve program performance. The baseline data for evaluation, collected in advance, can become a needs assessment instrument and influence the design of the program itself. Properly conceived, evaluation can lead to some understanding of *how* a program works, not just *that* it works. It can pinpoint the components of a complex design that can be sacrificed or must be maintained, if replication of an ambitious project has financial constraints more restrictive than those imposed on the experimental model. And it can assess the costs of the program, its cost-effectiveness and cost/benefit ratio, and can estimate the costs of replication.

In a climate of controversy or distrust, in times of financial constraint, in times that seek answers to troubling questions of public policy and program design, evaluation can play a significant role. This book does not seek to "teach" evaluation; that has been accomplished in many an excellent text. Rather it is a handbook on a particular model of evaluation in a particular setting, and it attempts to lead the reader step by step through the Scylla and Charybdis of evaluating a program in or in connection with schools and school systems. If it encourages administrators, providers, funders, and researchers to carry services to adolescents into a new generation of development, evaluation, program replication and redesign, it will serve its purpose.

Drawing on several years' experience with two schools involved in an intensive educational and service program and two schools that served as controls, this book will discuss what we found—and what others will, no doubt, find—when undertaking research in connection with school-based or school-linked programs. We will outline the *processes* involved in undertaking school-centered evaluation, *decisions* that need to be made at the outset, the *collection of data* on which measurement can be based, and a range of *technical and methodological problems* in the analysis of these data. Some of the issues addressed here will be specific to the assessment of programs in adolescent pregnancy prevention, but much of what we consider will apply equally well to other types of interventions that have to be evaluated in the school setting. Drug programs, sex education, smoking prevention and health promotion campaigns, and many other initiatives need to be evaluated in similar ways, in a setting where subjects move in, out, and through the system, where program exposure cannot necessarily be measured by enrollment, and where age is a critical variable. We will attempt to deal with the problems we had to solve in ways that will make our methodology useful in as wide as possible a range of programs, but we will focus, as well, on some of the particularly difficult variables that are specific to the field of reproductive health.

Choosing the Program to Evaluate

Not all projects are worthy of detailed, rigorous evaluation, nor do all programs need the same level of assessment. At a minimum, all programs owe their supporters and staff the assurance that they are doing what they set out to do; for that reason, we have tried to include suggestions for administrative review—the kinds of measurement providers can make themselves to keep track of their programs' effects. But, beyond that level of measurement, many programs are not so defined in their objectives nor so well staffed that they warrant full scale, academic review. How can one be reasonably certain that the evaluation will be worth the effort? The answer is not simple, since it involves the program's staff, its objectives, and the nature of the services themselves.

1. *Staff.* It takes courage to subject one's work to the scrutiny of outside researchers. However dedicated the staff, and however worthy the services, results may be far from the mark. It isn't every service provider who wants to find that out. Even with the will to know, the marriage between researcher and service staff is a difficult one at best. Shakespeare tells us misery makes strange bedfellows; so does evaluation. There needs to be real understanding on the part of the researcher of the risks the provider is taking, the time pressures on the program staff, the client or patient flow, the limits on paperwork, and the many problems of definition. On the other hand, the provider must make a commitment too: that honest data will be available, that staff will be properly oriented to that task, and that the demands of the researcher for information, once negotiated and delineated, will be met with accuracy and consistency. We will discuss these problems at some length, but list them here as minimal requirements when defining a useful setting for evaluation.

2. *Objectives.* There must be some agreement at the outset on the objectives of the program. Evaluation can only proceed in the light of defined purposes; without such definition, the selection of outcome measures is generally unsuccessful. If, for example, the governor's office has one set of objectives for a program, the local health department another, the school system yet another, and the program staff still another, it may be difficult to assess the overall success of the program. This does not mean that positive or negative effects cannot follow from services whether or not they were its primary goals; impacts often extend well beyond stated purposes. But, since the evaluator needs to know what outcomes are expected in order to select useful dependent variables, when there is no such agreement, a time-consuming evaluation may be premature. Does this mean that, without such political agreement, no assessments can be made? No, but at the very least, those who request the evaluation should be in a position to designate some set of outcome measures, whether or not all concerned with the program share

identical objectives. Nothing is more frustrating to researcher and provider alike than the discovery at the end of a long exercise that the researchers have been looking for outcomes the providers never sought to achieve!

3. *Services.* In turn, the services need to be related to the expected outcomes in such a way that there is a reasonable expectation the goals can be met. If, at first examination, such a clear relationship does not exist, that evidence alone could suggest a redefinition of long-term goals and short-term aims before an evaluation begins. Similarly, it is difficult to evaluate a program when many other services, quite outside the index project, are having their impact on the same population, at the same time. We will discuss this problem again, especially when we concentrate on the selection of adequate controls.

Thus, the very process of choosing an evaluator—or choosing a program to evaluate—can lead to useful change. From the outset, the relationship between the program staff and the research team can be revealing: if it is productive and cooperative, the decision to proceed with the evaluation can be a constructive move. If it feels like a confrontation, rather than a creative challenge, it may end up being a poor marriage indeed.

The Johns Hopkins Adolescent Pregnancy Prevention Program

What, then, was the program, the "marriage," upon which this review is based? We will describe it in some detail, so that references to the model throughout the text will be comprehensible. In our discussions, however, we will try to cover aspects of school-linked programs that differ from our model, since many such programs exist and many depart in substantive ways from that with which we were concerned when we developed this methodology. It is our hope that use of this material will not be limited to designs that share our model and/or its goals, but will extend to the evaluation of any educational, social, or medical intervention that uses the school as its population base.

The program under study was a primary pregnancy prevention program carried out in cooperation with the Baltimore City School System in an urban junior and senior high school. It was run by The Johns Hopkins School of Medicine, Departments of Pediatrics and of Gynecology/Obstetrics, with private funding for a three-year experimental intervention. It combined education, counseling, and medical services and operated both in the schools and in an adjacent clinic, with staff shared between the sites. A team consisting of a social worker and a nurse (practitioner or midwife) was assigned to each school. The social worker and, at times, the nurse were based in a health suite in their respective schools during the morning and through the lunch hour, available to faculty to give homeroom or classroom lectures, and available informally to the students for individual counseling, small group rap sessions, and educational encounters. No medical services were rendered in the school setting. Appointments could be made in school for clinic attendance in the afternoon; the clinic was open from early afternoon on for continued education and discussion and also for individual counseling and medical service, for males and females who thus became registered enrollees. Medical services included all types of reproductive health care—pregnancy tests, diagnosis and treatment of sexually transmitted diseases, and contraception. Diagnosis and referral for other health needs was routine, but the clinic was not billed as a comprehensive medical service; despite its storefront setting, it was a part of The Johns Hopkins Hospital network, which simplified the referral process.

The staff was a highly supportive, well-trained, and caring professional team. Its members, although nonjudgmental in their attitudes, put a great deal of emphasis on the development of value systems, on parental communication, and on responsible sexual conduct. They stressed the importance of making a life for oneself before making another life (hence the program's name, the Self Center). Although they made it clear that they did not believe early sexual onset to be in the students' best interests, and although they empowered students to say "no," they urged the use of contraception, instructed clients carefully in its use, and explained its importance at every coital act. Their counseling went way beyond the sexual realm, however, as they tried to help the students develop a set of goals and aspirations for their future achievement.

The staff were aware from the outset that the project involved evaluation, and were committed to the maintenance of accurate records, many of which involved detail that would not have been required under other circumstances. We shall discuss these several sources of data in subsequent chapters, and will comment on the ease or difficulty with which each type of information was collected.

As a condition for offering this program to the school system, it was made clear that data would have to be collected in the two program schools and in two control schools before the program began and at its close. In addition, information was gathered at two intermediate points in the program schools. The process of data collection by self-administered questionnaire within the school setting will be explored in the chapters that follow. The advantage of knowing, in advance, that a program is to be under careful scrutiny is immense. Although there are ways to evaluate programs without the collection of baseline data, the methodology developed here depends heavily on the availability of such information. For that reason, this text will be of greatest use to those who are designing new programs that will be evaluated; we trust it will be of some use, as well, to those who wish to evaluate programs already under way.

Use of the Text

This text will begin with an overall description of our evaluative design; it will discuss the choice of its quasi-experimental form, and will outline some of the difficulties in carrying out social research in a "real-world" situation. The review will proceed by describing data collection in a school setting, including the mechanics of data collection and such knotty questions as parental notification, anonymity, and dealing with the entire school community. We will discuss issues in the school population sample; these include questions of program exposure by grade and age, treatment of dropouts, absentees, and transfers, problems related to attendance and seasonal change, and the designation and use of control sites. The survey instrument will be described in some detail, including its range of knowledge, attitude and behavioral variables, reasons for their selection, and the process of cleaning and coding questionnaires, once collected. We will discuss the use of self-report in calculating rates of sexual activity, pregnancy, and program utilization. The study will proceed to address problems in the analysis of data, with an emphasis on methods of assessing change in key outcome measures. It will examine analytic methodologies. It will also address sources of data other than the self-administered questionnaire utilized in the school setting: these include detailed staff records, class records, and, last but not least, records from the clinic itself.

In each case, although largely drawn from the index program, we will use examples that illustrate the applicability of this methodology to other kinds of programs, especially other kinds of health interventions. Virtually all of the information we present will be equally adaptable to other outcome measures. The most complex case may well be the one we needed to address—the case of the pregnancy outcome; the methodology may, indeed, be more simply adapted to effects that are not time-related than it is to those with which we (and others interested in pregnancy prevention) are obliged to work.

A final word on the use of this book: Although we have described the program during whose evaluation the methodology was developed, this book is not "about" that model. It does not advocate one service model over another, nor does it argue for or against specific components of the project which proved so successful. What it does is to show how programs can be assessed overall, and makes a case for an evaluative design that can distinguish the effects of each major component of the program as well. This is because, in the real world, it is rare that a well-funded, experimental model can be replicated in full; the evaluation will be of most value if it can separate "necessary" components from those which, however well received, need not be reproduced.

In summary, this book can be used on many levels. It can suggest a general approach to the measurement of program effectiveness in the school setting; it can go a step further and propose some areas in which the service provider, with minimal research backup, can assess his or her own project; and it can be utilized by the applied researcher designing a rigorous, academic evaluation. Although it is in the last of those three processes that it will, no doubt, make its more important contribution, we will attempt, in each chapter, to indicate how to use the methodology on the simplest, as well as on the most technical, level.

Similarly, it is our hope that it will be of use to professionals with varying levels of experience in service provision and/or in evaluation. The health provider who has never worked in a school setting may find chapter 2 of interest, however well-versed in clinical evaluation. The experienced evaluator may never have encountered some of the special conditions of this age/grade-related context. If there are suggestions that appear too elementary to one reader, details that appear too technical to another, it is because we have tried to make our experience available to as varied an audience as possible in the multidisciplinary field we serve.

Most important, this work is based on the premise that there are no easy solutions to complex problems. There are, and will always be, elements of program effectiveness which elude measurement. However precise the methodology, there are human qualities that defy quantification, not the least of which is the willingness to engage our society's most solemn needs— and the courage to evaluate our success.

1
Evaluation Research: An Overview

Edward A. Smith

Evaluation within the Context of Program Development

Evaluation is one component of program development and diffusion. In this regard, program evaluation can serve multiple purposes. Obviously, of direct concern to an administrator, provider, or funding source is the question: Did it work? Of potentially equal importance, however, is the question: What did we learn so that we can improve upon the program or alter an existing one?

A multitude of programs currently exist to address the problems surrounding teen sexuality. These programs cover a broad range of intervention services including education, counseling, referral, pregnancy testing, and the provision of contraception. Unfortunately, although many of these programs are creative and achieve a great deal for the clients they serve, they often stand alone; sometimes they are short-lived and undocumented and thus may not contribute to the accumulating evidence offered by the successful and unsuccessful components of other programs. In such an environment, a field may constantly reinvent the wheel, and therefore do a poorer job, or a less efficient job, than it might.

Program evaluation, viewed from the broader context of program development, can move the field of teenage pregnancy prevention forward. In order to accomplish this objective, evaluations of programs must be methodologically sound and the results must be robust enough to withstand objective scrutiny. Although some may argue that evaluations are too costly, both in terms of time and funds, the alternative—a lack of knowledge regarding program efficacy and effectiveness—is significantly more costly in the long run. Of primary importance is the recognition that the evaluation of programs in a given field should be viewed along a developmental continuum: starting with some hypotheses as to what *might* work, developing the methods to test them, designing trials and studying them in defined populations, and finally demonstrating their success or failure and disseminating the results. Teenage pregnancy prevention is a field which has received increased attention over the past twenty-five years, but it is only beginning to move into the final two phases, testing and dissemination. Few demonstrations have been scientifically evaluated so they can be disseminated with confidence. Progress requires that we learn from our evaluations and refine new programs, so that we can move toward the goal of being able to diffuse programs of known effectiveness.

Types of Evaluation

There are many kinds of studies that fall under the general rubric of "evaluation." Although one may not *exclude* the other, they are conceptually different, and those who embark on this venture might well determine their real needs before setting out a research design.

As a first step, most evaluation research makes a distinction between "summative" and "formative" evaluation. Summative evaluation is used primarily at the *end* of a program to determine if goals and objectives have been met. Its primary objective is to determine the program's overall effectiveness and is often used as a benchmark against which success can be judged. Formative evaluation is an ongoing type of evaluation which measures progress during the *formation and implementation stages* of the program. Its primary purpose is to improve the program's effectiveness and to serve to feed back information to providers at interim stages in the life of the program. Often, administrators, policymakers, and upper-level managers make use of summative evaluation, whereas formative evaluation is often most useful to those who develop and implement programs.

It is important to note that any instrument or technique can be both formative and summative depending upon how it is used. Sound evaluation of teenage pregnancy prevention programs should utilize both summative and formative evaluation methods. To illustrate a formative program evaluation technique, the program at Johns Hopkins provided information, on an intermittent basis, to the program staff in order to help improve program delivery. Following each spring survey (to be discussed later), the research staff met with the clinical staff to review preliminary data. Included in these discussions were the students' anonymous reports of their likes and dislikes or their use and details of use of various program components. When feasible, program modifications, using this information, were implemented to improve program delivery and acceptance. The same surveys provided the data for summative research: the determination of the actual effects of the program's services at the end of the experimental period.

In addition to summative and formative evaluation, M.Q. Patton (in *Utilization Focused Evaluation.* Beverly Hills: Sage Publications, 1978) conceptualizes three other types of evaluation that are applicable to teen programs: "effort" evaluation, "process" evaluation, and "treatment specification" evaluation. Effort evaluation represents an assessment of input or energy, regardless of the output. Such measures include staff time; staff to client ratio; spending on space, materials, or equipment; and problems relating to these factors. In sum, effort evaluation usually involves making an inventory of program operations. In many instances, dollar costs can be a straightforward manner in which to assess and compare effort across programs.

Process evaluation focuses on the internal dynamics and actual operations of a program in an attempt to understand its successes, as well as barriers to success, and changes in the program. Indices to be used in process evaluation include perceptions of the clients and their informal patterns of behavior, unanticipated consequences, a sequencing of activities and an understanding of how program activities are coordinated. Process evaluation is usually developmental, descriptive, continuous, flexible, and inductive. It requires sensitivity to both quantitative and qualitative data. It is of particular importance to those who come later and want to replicate parts or all of a successful program. Research which tells them that given inputs produced given outputs, but gives them no information on *what was actually done*, makes replication difficult and often leaves program designers in the dark.

A number of methods of process evaluation can be applied to teen pregnancy programs. Qualitatively, for example, focus groups may provide valuable insight into factors which may influence program acceptance and adherence. Staff can give detailed descriptions of their activities. Ideally, qualitative data can be supplemented with quantitative data to understand the *process* by which the program worked. Under these circumstances, qualitative information can help in both framing the right questions and structuring the range of potential answers; quantitative data, in turn, should reflect the *degree* to which these processes exist within the population. Questions which might be addressed in process evaluation include: What did the staff *do?* How did the teen learn of the program? What specifically motivated the teen to come to the clinic? Why did he or she choose a specific method? How did the staff get the teen to return? In sum, process evaluation asks the question "How did it work?"

Treatment specification evaluation addresses three essential questions: (1) What are the specific program features which caused the observed effect? (2) How sensitive are the measurement instruments? Can they detect the program's effects? (3) Under what conditions (that is, when? where? how? with whom?) could we expect to see the effects? Treatment specification evaluation involves a critical analysis and a precise identification of what it is about a program that is supposed to have an effect. Unfortunately, evaluations are often not successful because they do not ask questions that are precise enough to reflect program impact. For example, in evaluating school-linked pregnancy programs, we need to get information on sequences of events; that is, on the relative timing of events that are of programmatic interest. A question which asks, for example, "Have you *ever* been pregnant?" does not provide a time reference which can be juxtaposed with the existence of the program. Likewise, asking a girl if she has had a birth, an abortion, or a miscarriage in the last twelve months can also be misleading—the conception associated with such events may be as little as one month, or as long as twenty-one months, ago!

The specification of treatment effects underscores the need to tie the treatment (program) to its outcomes. Contraceptive behavior, for example, should be linked to the services available. If a clinic is provided, the behavior of clinic attendees should be contrasted with those who did not attend. Likewise, an analysis of participation in other components of a program should be conducted. The objective should be the identification of key elements which discriminate between components of a program which were conducive to (or were perhaps obstacles to) successful outcomes.

Each of these five types of evaluation is important and can provide a wealth of information about a program's success and the manner in which it operated. Ideally, a comprehensive evaluation will involve components of each type; realistically, compromises will have to be made regarding the resources used in the evaluation effort. In planning an evaluation, however, researchers and/or providers must critically and objectively assess the ability of their research plans to measure their program's impact.

Methods of Evaluative Research

There exist a number of methods for conducting the forms of evaluative research discussed in the preceding. These methods range from historical and case analysis to the execution of true experimental designs involving the random assignment of treatment and control groups. Often, however, the inherent nature of the problem, costs, opportunities, or policy decisions will have an impact on the nature of the research design. True experimental designs, for example, may be extremely difficult in a human context. They are rare in social research. This is certainly true in the field of adolescent pregnancy prevention: the advantages of random assignment to treatment and control groups must be weighed against the ethical consideration of withholding services (either services whose effects are not yet firmly established or services like family planning whose benefits are clear) from those who may need them. Indeed, one rarely has the opportunity for such an experimental design, in any case.

The field of adolescent pregnancy research is not unique in facing this applied research dilemma. The use of quasi-experimental designs takes into account the fact that in most social situations the choice of the treatment group is not entirely random. Furthermore, it recognizes that the control groups will probably not be from precisely the same populations as the treatment groups. This means, for example, that although background characteristics such as race, age, and completed education should be as close as possible, initial levels of outcome measures such as pregnancy rates, contraceptive behavior, sexual activity, cigarette smoking, or alcohol consumption may be somewhat different in the two groups. When such conditions exist, a "non-equivalent control group" design is employed. "Non-equivalent" should not imply that one can use any control group one can find; the attempt must be to find the best available match. It merely suggests that if there are minor variations, that need not destroy the usefulness of the control.

Critical to the use of such a design, however, is the acquisition of pre-test (or pre-program) data from both groups. This pre-program information, in combination with post-program information, allows not only for the evaluation of change in the group receiving the program, but also provides information on historical or secular trends by monitoring change during the same period in the group *not* receiving the program.

The Johns Hopkins Research Program

The research protocol used to evaluate the Johns Hopkins Pregnancy Prevention Program was a quasi-experimental, non-equivalent control group design. The five basic types of evaluation research (summative, formative, effort, process, treatment specification) previously discussed were all employed in a comprehensive evaluation whose methods will be presented in this book. The initial summative evaluation appears as appendix A.

The Design

Two schools, a junior and senior high school, were selected by project and school officials to receive the program for a number of practical reasons, such as proximity to The Johns Hopkins Hospital and the desire of their principals to take part. Another junior and senior high school, as similar as possible in some identifiable ways, were recruited to serve as controls.

Figure 1–1 is an overview of the research timetable as it was conducted in both the treatment and the control schools. In addition to the data collection points, this figure displays the introduction of the two major components of the intervention: school services and the program clinic.

Surveys were conducted in the two program schools during the fall of program year one *prior to the introduction of either component of the program*. These data, collected by self-administered questionnaire, served as pre-program, baseline information. The same questionnaire was administered in

	School Year One		School Year Two		School Year Three	
	Fall	Spring	Fall	Spring	Fall	Spring
Program	School component ———————————————————————————→					
	Clinic component ————————————————————————————→					
Program Schools:						
Senior high	Q	Q		Q		Q
Junior high	Q	Q		Q		Q
Control Schools:						
Senior High	Q					Q
Junior High	Q					Q
	$time_1$	$time_2$		$time_3$		$time_4$

Note: Q = Questionnaire (self-administered)

Figure 1–1. Overview of Research Timetable

the control schools during the same school year in which it was administered in the program schools. At the end of the first school year, a readministration of the questionnaire was conducted in the program schools; it was repeated again at the end of the second school year. In all four schools, program and control, the survey was administered at the end of the third program year, when the program terminated.

It should be noted that data from the program schools (that is, the experimental group) were collected at *four* different points; in the non-program schools (that is, the control group), data were only collected *twice*. This research design was efficient, and still was able to serve two essential purposes: (1) it allowed us to discover whether there were secular changes during the three-year period of the program by comparing the baseline to follow-up data from the control schools, and (2) it captured subsets of the adolescents exposed to the program's services before they exited from the experimental schools. For example, at the end of program year one, all of the twelfth-grade students in the senior high and the majority of the ninth-grade students in the junior high exited the program schools (that is, they graduated). Without the spring data collection at the end of year one in the program schools, we would have "lost" the ability to measure program effects on these two groups. Likewise, spring data collection at the end of program year two captured the same graduating subset (that is, the twelfth-grade students in the senior high and the ninth-grade students in the junior high). This complicated question of program exposure will be dealt with in further detail in chapter 3, since it is a critical part of our evaluation design.

The interim surveys in the program schools also permitted program information to be fed back to the staff, and allowed for the preliminary assessment of change. The former purpose was served, as mentioned previously, when the surveys provided formative evaluation data for the program staff. The latter purpose was met when surveys were used to see whether or not there were early indicants of the program's intended effects. Thus, although collected for purposes of evaluation, the questionnaires helped to modify program delivery in years two and three.

The basic model, then, consists of the comparison of "before" and "after" in the program and the non-program schools, with the *direction of change* and the *magnitude of change* within each population as the basic measurement of interest. Chapter 3 will detail the overall evaluation strategy, the effects of choosing the entire student bodies of the four schools as the sample of interest, and the use and limits of control populations. The choice of the entire school population is basic to our model. It is based on the premise that initiatives that target schools should be measured by their ability to reach that entire target group. Since school-linked programs are often justified by citing their ability to reach those who might never attend less accessible clinics, and by their ability to educate even those who do not seek out education, it seems logical to monitor these initiatives' ability to reach all the students in their target schools. Aggregate information on program utilization is built into the survey, so that the relationship between variables of interest and individual (anonymous) characteristics can also be assessed; groups who utilized one or another service can be separately analyzed when the value of specific components of service is being reviewed. However, the evaluation's first concern is the program's impact on the school as a whole. Since the duration of program exposure differs by grade, and since program effects may differ by age, the model controls for grade and exposure in assessing change. It develops summary measures incorporating those controls in order to report effects at the aggregate level.

Other portions of the evaluation rely on data sources that go far beyond the surveys of the student populations. These sources, described in chapter 6, allow the researchers to explore such areas as the cost-effectiveness of the program, the utilization of its component parts, and the effects of clinic attendance. Basic to all of these, however, is the model outlined previously, because if the outcomes are not reliably measured, and if they do not prove that the program was overall a success, the costs of its inputs or the evaluation of specific intervention elements are of little academic or professional importance. How, then, can we be certain that the evaluation is an accurate assessment of program effects?

Dealing with Validity

As with any program evaluation, the program discussed here had to address questions of both internal and external validity. External validity is the ability to generalize the findings to other settings and to repeat them in similar settings. This is limited by the degree to which one believes one's population (defined here as an inner-city, black, low-income population) is the same as or different in other characteristics of interest from other populations similarly defined. Whatever limits one places on the generalizability of the study, however, they do not call into question the *method* employed in the evaluation: the method discussed here should be equally valid in other settings.

Internal validity involves the linkage between cause and effect: if a change is observed, can we attribute the change to the program? Internal validity is of primary interest in applied social research; observations of covariation and a proper time sequence of events are necessary, but not sufficient, conditions for causality. For example, had we known *only* that pregnancy rates decreased and contraceptive use increased in the treatment schools during the Hopkins program, it could not automatically have been assumed that these changes were all due to the program. At a minimum, the absence of a similar change in the control schools was required before this conclusion could be reached. The focus of much research effort, and an important role of the control group, is to check internal validity—to ensure that the observed change, positive or negative, is attributable to the intervention effort.

There are many factors that can threaten the internal validity of a study such as this, some of which are inherent in the nature of an evaluation of different age groups over time, some of which have to do with "historical" events which may intervene with a study population, and some of which have to do with the sample—its size, its potential for change over time, selectivity biases, and so on. Based on the Hopkins experience, a few examples will suggest how well one must know the program, its participants, and its staff, to be certain that no such contamination occurs.

1. In comparing schools that have, to those that do not have, an experimental program, is one certain no new initiative was undertaken in the control schools or the program schools during the experimental period? Did something change in the environment of the schools—a new clinic in the neighborhood, a change in the curriculum? By keeping in close touch with all four schools, the danger of missing such contamination was avoided. This potential problem should be of particular concern to researchers who are not in immediate or ongoing contact with their study populations.

2. Did students have a choice between program exposure and no program exposure? Were there different kinds of people in the schools? Could selectivity have biased the study? In the Hopkins case, where entire schools formed the populations of interest, there was no such selectivity problem. Whether or not particular students in the program schools took part at one or another level does, indeed, reflect individual differences, differences which tell a great deal about the program and how it worked. However, the essential comparison on which the evaluation is based, between change in the

experimental and change in the control groups, must not be based on people who chose versus people who chose not to participate.

3. Did the measurement instruments stay the same over time? Chapter 4 addresses this question, and underlines the importance of consistency in survey design.

4. Did different types of people get lost to follow-up in the experimental versus the control schools? Dropouts, transfers, refusals would all have an effect if not closely monitored. Chapter 3 explains the methods used to be as certain as possible that no such contamination occurs.

5. How does one manage the maturing of the population over time? Those exposed to a program are older after exposure than they were before—how can one be certain the changes over time are not due to the aging process alone? The use of individual grades as the unit of comparison will be explained in chapter 3; in combination with specific years of program exposure, the problem of maturation is minimized.

As should be clear from these examples, some threats to the validity of an evaluation are inherent in the nature of the population—in this case, an age- /grade-controlled, in-school student sample—and thus will apply to *any* school-linked intervention. Others require intimate contact with the program of interest, and may apply in only one specific setting. We will address both types of problems in the course of this discussion, because even the "special" cases may serve to alert the reader to some potential problem that lies in wait.

In addition to these threats to internal validity and the need, in the long run, to question generalizability, researchers must be concerned with problems of "statistical conclusion" validity (for example, power, sample size, levels of significance) and "construct validity" (that is, measurement issues). The ability to make conclusive statements is often a function of these two factors. Inadequate sample sizes, especially when tied to poor measurement instruments, may lead one to conclude that there was no effect even in a highly successful program.

It is important to note that trade-offs are often involved when researchers address the technical problems and the multiple purposes of program evaluation. Applied research in an area such as pregnancy prevention will be most useful if it assigns clear priorities to its research design, so that it reflects local needs on the one hand, and on the other, helps to effect social change by advancing knowledge in the field. The evaluation design for the Hopkins program, for example, needed to serve several ends. In this case, the local goals were quite clear and of prime importance: to reduce adolescent pregnancy, by postponing sexual onset, if possible, and by increasing contraceptive use among the sexually active. These goals were paralleled by the need to execute and design objective, dependable, and replicable research to serve the larger field. These twin objectives resulted in a concern for a scientific balance between high internal validity (that is, being able to attribute change to the program), high construct validity (that is, assuming that measures properly assessed knowledge, attitudes, and behavior), and precise, practical statistical analyses.

The resulting evaluation model requires the collection of many data sets; those used in the Hopkins study will be described in chapters 4 and 6. It requires aggregate information on the student bodies gleaned from school questionnaires. It also requires documentation of the day-to-day activities of the staff and their daily contacts with the students. How detailed these sets are will be up to each provider/evaluator team to decide. The decisions of the researchers with respect to these data sets are translated, first, into survey design, and then into an analytic methodology. Most important, the model requires close cooperation with the schools themselves, which will be the focus of the next chapter.

2

Collecting Data in a School Context

T here are few institutions as complicated to work with as public schools, not because they are deliberately resistant—often they are individually cordial and receptive—but because of the nature of the systems in which they operate. Principals may appear at first glance to operate independently, in fiefdoms of their own. However, although they are sometimes in a position to *reject* new programs or relationships, they are rarely permitted to *accept* them without the approval of an arcane network of boards, committees, regional supervisors, departmental officers, and administrative authorities. School systems in the United States have a tradition of community jurisdiction and parental involvement, complicated by their official responsibility to local government, by their relationships with teachers' organizations, and by their accountability to the public, the media, and, in fact, to anyone or any agency which demands that accountability. They cannot move quickly and can rarely move easily. Even when they are anxious to cooperate, there is "process" to be observed—process which one is at peril to ignore.

Since the schools are often hard pressed in the current financial climate for the funds for special services they feel their students need, those agencies that can come to principals with an offer of staff or service are more welcome than those that come asking only for favors. Administering the surveys on which the present model depends is such a "favor." This is another argument for building evaluation into programs from the outset, because the request for data collection can then be made as a part of a service package the principal is anxious to receive. The process is reciprocal, and both parties gain from it. Even when a survey *is* a part of a larger program, however, it should be understood that the privilege of collecting data in a school setting is a favor for the school to grant—one that places demands upon the entire school community.

Why would the process be seen as beneficial by the school administration? A schoolwide survey can be seen on the first level as a risk assessment tool, describing the needs of the particular student body for particular types of services. Its results can help the principal to explain or, if necessary, to justify the special program to parent groups and others who may question it. Second, it can be seen as an educational device, informing the students in a very concrete way of the scope of the program which will be undertaken, permitting them to report (albeit anonymously) on behaviors they may never have discussed with adults, and suggesting that these are legitimate areas to explore with the professionals who will be available to them. Finally, the survey is valued for its basic purpose: a conscientious principal is anxious to know whether or not a program, offered selectively to certain schools, is truly effective. Use of the information as baseline data for a serious evaluation is understood and appreciated as a correlate of the service program.

Why, then, would a non-program school be willing to take part as a "control"? For parallel reasons, with a different twist. As an assessment tool, the data can help communities, principals or superintendents of entire school systems to understand their school populations, and may, in fact, be the means by which they will attract the programs they require. At the very least, the data may help make a case for students' needs which an administrator has already identified, but has heretofore been unable to document. Thus, those responsible for student populations in areas where no special services are as yet available may wish to participate as a step in the needs assessment and planning process.

The researcher who wishes to administer a schoolwide survey must begin by understanding the magnitude of the task he or she is asking the principal to undertake. On the functional level it is a task involving the logistics of administration, which we will discuss in the following. But before taking on that task, the principal must make several tactical decisions, with one or another level of supervision by the superintendent of the school system. These decisions include the orientation of faculty and of parents: How much explanation? How much orientation? Should it be in the nature of consultation or should it seek advice and consent? Should it be face-to-face or in writing? Should it be in committee or in general meeting? How much information should the students receive prior to administration of a questionnaire? What kind of parental notification should be required? The answers to some of these questions may actually impinge on the study itself, as they affect the quality of the students' response. However, they will relate primarily to the principals' personal styles, to the school systems in which they operate, to the strength of the parents' and teachers' organizations within their schools, and to other relationships beyond the control of the research team. Whatever the principal, or the principal's surrogate, proposes as a modus operandi will probably be essential to the success of the project, because no survey can be carried out without complete administrative support.

As the foregoing makes clear, this discussion might well have been called "The Politics of Data Collection," and, as with politics in any area, it is well to understand the legitimate interests and concerns of those with whom one is working. What are some of the issues that affect their decisions in the areas we have listed?

First, there is the image of the school, the perception the community has of the school both as representative of the community and as a reflection of the families and/or the school system it represents. The principal and the superintendent of schools have a strong interest in protecting that image, and need some guarantees that the data, labeled by school, will not appear in the press and in some way suggest that the student population is aberrational, inferior, ill-behaved, or deficient. These assurances must be given, but with the caveat that, however well the research team observes its promises, there can be slips when the media get involved. Every effort needs to be made to protect the data, and not to allow it to be quoted irresponsibly some months or years down the line.

Second is the perception of the parents and the community of the selection of *their* children, *their* neighborhood, as the "guinea pig." They have every right to be somewhat defensive. They need explanation and reassurance, and may need to be involved in the planning process. Community leaders, parents, and clergy will be supportive only in proportion to their understanding of the true purpose of the endeavor; that takes time, and as one researcher has put it, "standing naked before them."

A third issue is the ownership and use of the data. Does the research exploit the student body for the researchers' purposes, or does it really benefit the schools directly? Is is organized so it *can* benefit them, and are questions which they see as relevant included? Will they have access to the data? Should they? How can cooperative agreements be engineered that would protect the interests of the providers, the researchers, and the school system?

Fourth, will the decision to take part in the study affect teacher-administration relationships, parent-school relationships, interdepartmental relationships? There are questions of turf to be defended. For example, will the science and health faculty feel threatened or, indeed, will their area of interest be strengthened? How do school nurses feel about the study—does it appear to them to "judge" their performance or does it lend them support? What about guidance counselors? Or teachers in areas not, apparently, related? Can the moral objections of one popular faculty member, for example, affect school attitudes toward the study? Will that, in turn, affect attitudes toward the program under evaluation?

Fifth, to carry that last question one step further, what will be the perceived relationship between the study and the program itself? If the evaluation is seen as a *risk* to the program rather than a contributing part of it, then that perception could adversely affect answers to all the issues raised here. Is it worth embarking on the study if, indeed, it does? How can one avoid that negative perception?

Clearly, these are legitimate concerns. The only generic advice is that careful observation of the school systems' "process," careful attention to negotiated protocols, and careful orientation of the many constituencies involved requires thoughtful cooperation between the school, the program administrators, and the researchers—and in some cases, parents and communities as well. The more bases covered in advance, the more supporters within the schools with a stake in its success, the better the project's chances. On the other hand, if after that is accomplished there remains vocal objection on the part of a small group of unreconciled opponents, however loud that objection may be, perhaps it should be ignored; the generally positive support most of these endeavors have received should not be threatened by a tiny minority. With cautious preparation, the school community will probably share that perception.

Issues in Survey Administration

Once these issues are resolved, the process can move on to the administration of a baseline questionnaire. This involves (l) decisions on parental notification; (2) decisions on the orientation of faculty; (3) protection of anonymity and voluntarism; and (4) the mechanics of administration itself.

Parental Notification

The nature of the questions that are required to provide the baseline for evaluation of programs in such sensitive areas as pregnancy, substance use, and other adolescent problems makes it likely that most school systems will want some measure of parental contact to precede survey administration. This can range from requiring written consent from parents for the participation of their offspring, through sharing the questionnaire with parents upon request, to parental notification only. Clearly, the requirement of *notification only* is very much to the advantage of the research because (l) it makes for maximal participation in the survey and (2) it makes for a minimum of discussion of the instrument itself before its administration. Getting written consent is not only a cumbersome process but results in a nonrandom selection of participants and would call the results into serious question. It may even reduce the numbers so far that the data are useless. Every attempt should be made to avoid it.

On the other hand, it is altogether proper that parents know of the activity and have the opportunity to withdraw their sons and daughters from participation should they so desire. Fortunately, experience suggests that few will do so. Either the researchers or the principal can handle the notification and exemption process, but the letter of notification should, ideally, come out over the principal's signature. It is usually a familiar name to the school family, and a trusted one, and the principal's leadership role underlines the integration of the activity into the school program.

What should the notification include? (See appendix B.) Preferably the *reason* for the survey, the *concern* of the faculty for the well-being of the student body, the *seriousness* of the problem(s) the program will address, and the *voluntary and anonymous* nature of the survey itself. If the survey covers areas already treated in the school curriculum, it will minimize parental concern if that fact is noted. Finally, it should include a number to call, preferably the principal's, should they wish further information, or should they want their offspring exempt from the survey program.

Orientation of Faculty

The faculty, by their attitudes toward the project, can have a major effect on its success or failure. Time invested in working with them is extremely well spent. If the faculty will be involved in handing out the questionnaires and monitoring the students during its administration, they must know what they are doing and why. The amount of their involvement will not only depend on the style of the principal, as mentioned previously, but on the number of research and/or service staff from the program available to assist in the process.

Meetings with faculty will not be discussed here because, as useful as such meetings are, they are best managed by the principal or his or her delegate. The research staff and the service staff can and should be available to explain the program, but should not be called upon to tell the teachers their role. They should be present to answer the faculty's questions, however, to describe the forthcoming administration of the survey, and to play any part required of them by the principal.

Whether or not such meetings are held, however, the research staff *is* responsible for the preparation of extensive and carefully written instructions for monitoring the survey. In writing the teachers' memo, one should be sensitive to the fact that public school faculty often view with alarm *any* additions to their accepted, defined functions. Their cooperation cannot be taken for granted; they should be thanked for their participation before they are led through the process, step by step. Discussion of the process must include which surveys (by color, number, or whatever identification mark is used) go to whom; how to orient the students; the actual words to read to the students to explain the anonymous and voluntary nature of the study; the fact that it is a survey, *not* a test; the timetable for the survey process; and the method to be used for tallying and collecting the surveys so that teachers will not handle individual completed forms. This last subject is important, and can involve having the students place the completed forms in an envelope or box on the teacher's desk, unless they are collected directly by a member of the research staff. Our teachers' memo ended with repeated thanks for what the faculty might well see as a major interruption of their academic schedules.

Confidentiality, Anonymity, and Student Consent

Students, as well as their parents, need to be assured of the privacy of their response. They need to believe the promise of anonymity; that entails telling them *not* to sign their questionnaires, explaining that coding numbers, if any appear on the forms, are not unique numbers and cannot identify them as individuals, and arranging a method of survey collection that makes it impossible for their teachers to look at their responses. It is well to recall that some of the questions to which they are asked to respond are self-incriminating, and perhaps even involve confessions that have legal implications (for example, fatherhood and hard drug use). Without a real belief in the system set up for their protection, it would be irrational for them to respond honestly. Given that assurance, however, teenagers are generally at an altruistic age, and will be more than willing to help their contemporaries if that is what they believe honest response to the survey will accomplish.

They also need to know that participation is voluntary, that even accepting the questionnaire and starting to fill it out does not commit them to answering any question they prefer to skip, nor even prevent them from stopping half way through it. Refusal rates should still be low, when anonymity is also assured. In fact, their understanding that they may discontinue their participation *after* accepting the questionnaire may actually lead to greater acceptance of the survey in the first place. Students may be less hesitant to take it, and to begin filling it out, if they know they still have options left them; once they begin, it is rare that the forms are too incomplete to be of use.

The assurances of anonymity and voluntary participation can best be accomplished in three ways: first, through the parental notification letter; second, through an announcement made by the teacher or other survey administrator when the forms are distributed; and third, through a paragraph printed on the top of the instrument itself. The administrator should also be carefully briefed, so that individual questions in the classroom receive the appropriate response.

Some researchers have attempted to collect similar data using a numerical identifier so that longitudinal analysis is possible. In this case, a cover sheet associating the student's name and number is filled out, torn off and retained on a confidential basis by the researchers. Only the number is on the questionnaire itself, and only the number appears in the computer file. Although this method does not guarantee anonymity, but does promise some measure of confidentiality, it is reported to have excellent acceptance. It requires that the name and number be linked again in future, when the follow-up questionnaires are administered.

The number-linked method was not used in the Hopkins study. The schools preferred true anonymity; they were content with a negative parental consent procedure, which they would not have considered sufficient had the students been identifiable. The researchers elected total anonymity for the students too, even though it prohibited a panel study, because the students' clear preference for anonymity made it appear that any kind of identification technique could endanger the reliability of their response. Given the choice between quality of data and longitudinal design, we opted for the data, since a longitudinal design could be approximated by comparing aggregate data at different points in time. Others may wish to weigh this choice for themselves.

Where to Administer the Survey

Several plans have been used to assure coverage of the entire student body (or whatever subset is selected should a sample be taken). The plan advocated here utilizes the homeroom to which each student is assigned. Using the homeroom has several advantages over other administration plans which have been tried, especially when the school's schedule specifies homeroom attendance in the first period: (1) All students have a homeroom assignment; (2) teachers have relatively good, up-to-date lists of their homeroom students and are generally responsible to the school for accounting for their attendance; (3) students are less likely to "cut" homeroom, since it is there that attendance is taken; (4) teachers can be asked to pick up the survey instruments and their instructions as they arrive in the morning, or can have them delivered to the classroom while students congregate, without interfering with a preceding class; (5) the entire process is accomplished early in the day, at one time for everyone. Thus, it is less disruptive, more time efficient, and there is no occasion for the students to compare notes, discuss questions, or in any other way contaminate their individual response before some have completed the survey.

Other methods of administration which have been tried include selecting a class that all students have each day (for example, English) and administering the survey when students attend that class, or bringing the students into the auditorium so that more can be handled by a smaller research team. The disadvantages of each of these methods are apparent. The former means that each group receives the questionnaire at a different time of day, maximizing hallway "buzzing" and discussion, and probably reducing the numbers who participate. The latter process is difficult to control. It further reduces the number of participants, since many will be lost en route from the class to the auditorium; any time students are moved, some stragglers will disappear. What is worse, those lost will probably represent a nonrandom sample—perhaps even the subset one would most like to reach. The homeroom method, or failing that, the first period in the morning whatever it is, is probably the safest plan.

One final caution: if the first period is used for the survey, all students should be directed to their first period classrooms even if they arrive late. (The same procedure should apply at whatever time of day the survey is administered.) The questionnaires should be designed to take less than an entire class period to allow for instructions, handing out the forms, and so on. Latecomers can often complete the survey without any trouble.

Response Rates: Refusals and Absentees

With optimal preparation, and with parental notification in lieu of consent, there is every reason to believe that levels of student participation will be high. It was not unusual to achieve a 98 percent response rate among students present on the day of administration. Included in the 2 percent refusal rate are the occasional student whose parent requested exemption, and the few students in the classrooms who elected not to complete the questionnaire.

In order to count refusals accurately, the teachers in the Hopkins study were told to hand out questionnaires to each student in the room. Each teacher had a packet containing the numbers of male and female forms required for their registered students, and each packet was labeled with the number of male and female questionnaires enclosed. Teachers were responsible for returning that number at the end of the period. A simple check sheet completed by the teacher could then account for his or her correct tally:

$$\text{Total} = \text{Absentees} + \text{Refusals} + \text{Completions}$$

(Occasionally, teachers reported that the numbers given us as the numbers of registered students in their homerooms were not correct. They almost always reported that our number was too high, not too low. These differences may represent dropouts during the interval since the school lists were drawn up.) By maintaining a rigid count, several objectives were served.

1. Refusal rates could be computed using the actual number present as the denominator.

2. A revised count of registered students in the schools could be calculated.

3. A preliminary count of completed forms could be made.

4. All the forms were brought back to the research team. We considered it of utmost importance that blank questionnaires not circulate in the com-

munity, not because parents who wished to see them could not ask to do so, but because familiarity with the forms could affect other schools in the study, or readministration in the school itself.

Note that the 98 percent response rate previously mentioned is qualified by the phrase "among students present on the day of administration." In public schools throughout the United States, absentees represent a considerable proportion of the student body. Attendance may be in the 80 percent range, at times even lower. In chapter 3 we will discuss the handling and the possible effects of this sad phenomenon on the study, but we note the problem here because an administrative decision will have to be made as to whether or not to conduct the survey on more than one day. To the extent that absenteeism represents true illness, or was particularly high on the day of administration, a considerable proportion can be picked up by repeating the survey the next week, with the principal's approval. The principal will have to arrange that any students present on the second date, who were absent on the first date, be sent from their classrooms to a central area designated for the survey. Since the repeat performance may be seen as disruptive, and since it is unlikely that it will pick up chronic absentees, the researchers might comfortably opt for a single survey day.

Special Education Classes

The problem of administering a written questionnaire to youngsters with limited reading skills is a pervasive challenge in school-based survey design. Age-graded instruments are necessary even for students who function at or close to grade level, but these instruments may not answer the more difficult problems of slow readers or students in special education classes. Nonetheless, some means of including these students should be found, because by excluding them, valuable information may be lost. The correlation between low school achievement and such problems as premature termination of schooling, early pregnancy, and low self-esteem suggest, not surprisingly, that this selected group should be a part of any meaningful study.

Once in a senior high school, students who have been promoted to this level should be able to read the questionnaire if it has been properly designed. However, if middle or junior high school students are in the study, the combination of youth and especially low reading skills may make it necessary to adapt the administration process to their special needs. In the Hopkins study, good results were obtained by using the same instrument, completed individually and anonymously by each student, but read out loud, question by question, by one of the survey team. Students were divided into male and female classrooms for this purpose, and a same-sex individual administered the survey during the same homeroom period. Best results are obtained if the principal makes a little extra time available, because moving the students and explaining the process take time, and the reading must be slow. Since the questionnaire is completed in the same way as it is by other students, there is no reason to believe the results are not valid once questions are heard and understood. Of course, instruments can be numbered by classroom (see chapter 4) so these special cases can be separately examined during the analysis phase, if desired. However, to achieve a picture of the entire school's student population, results obtained from these classrooms should be analyzed with all of the rest of the questionnaires.

Creating an Atmosphere of Cooperation

The steps outlined in the preceding sections should help create an atmosphere in which the students, faculty, and administration work hand in hand for the good of the project. In the long run, it is a positive constructive relationship between the research staff, the program staff, and the principal that makes the survey "work." Some specific examples may illustrate the process on the day itself:

1. Representatives of the survey team need to be present at administration, to guide, monitor, and support the school's faculty. Since there are rarely enough researchers to man all the sites in the school, the program's staff can be utilized, as well, and the team judiciously apportioned to lend a hand where they are needed. In the Hopkins case, each member of the research and program team had assigned classrooms (usually four or five) to cover. Each made personal contact with the classroom teacher to check that the questionnaires were in hand, that the directions were clear, and to answer last minute questions. Each returned to his or her assigned classrooms several times during the hour to ask the students if they had questions of their own. Each was responsible for picking up unused questionnaires (absences, refusals) late in the hour and, finally, each was responsible for picking up completed questionnaires at the end of the survey.

2. Of particular concern were classrooms with substitute teachers—all too common in the public school system. These teachers generally have much less authority in their homerooms than the regular faculty, and have almost certainly received little or no orientation about the survey activity. They need to be identified early in the morning, and the surveyors who are assigned to their classrooms need to be available most of the time, when they are not making their calls to other homeroom posts.

3. It should not be assumed that all teachers will cooperate with the survey team to the same degree. One may not wish to read material as written, another may wish to handle students without the team's involvement, and it is even possible that an occasional teacher may discourage the students from participating. This is rare, and if the principal has done a good

job of orientation, should not happen. The only recourse of the team on the day of the survey is to the principal or the principal's surrogate; there is neither time nor an appropriate manner of handling these situations directly without risking the future of the program. Better yet, be sure the groundwork has been laid so these aberrations do not occur.

4. Some schools, especially large public high schools, are so impersonal and vast that one-to-one contact is difficult. Often these schools have public address systems, which are used for early morning announcements on a regular basis. Principals often use them to urge students to their classrooms at the opening bell, or to lead them in the pledge of allegiance. A cooperative principal can make that system available to the research director to address the entire school family with a few words about the importance of their participation, with last minute instructions, and with thanks. The atmosphere for a truly cooperative effort is established when the principal introduces the researchers, and when the researchers reach out to commend the students on their contribution.

These are but a few ways that the team effort can be strengthened. Each new setting should suggest its own, once a true partnership has been forged.

Simplifying the Data Collection Process

Reading our description of survey administration, the question, "Can one simplify the survey data collection process, and if so, how?" is bound to occur. Unfortunately, there are few compromises that can be suggested, and none that diminish the major investment of time spent in laying the groundwork for fruitful cooperation. To short-circuit that process would, in the long run, be self-defeating.

Once good relationships are established, there is one simple alternative to the time-consuming method of survey administration we describe, and that is to have the schools handle it themselves. It would not be advisable to remove all contact with the schools on "survey day"; at least one or two research/provider representatives should be on the scene. But the team of researchers we describe, monitoring clusters of classrooms and coordinating the effort, can be replaced by school personnel if their orientation by program and research staff has been thorough. Of course, that process, in itself, takes time.

Another accommodation might be to reduce data collection to the beginning and end of the experimental period in the program schools as we did in the controls. This would entail omitting the surveys at the end of intervening years. Disadvantages include (1) loss to the study of graduates in the intervening years; (2) inability to feed interim data back to the program staff; (3) heavy reliance on the final administration of the survey (that is, if any problems arise, the entire study is at risk); and (4) inability to measure trends or to determine an expected timetable for change. Advantages may include not only a large saving in time for data collection, management, and analysis, but a lower risk of "surfeiting" the students with an overload of questions at too frequent intervals.

There will, inevitably, be compromises along the way. Things will happen on the day of administration for which no one is prepared. Whatever methods are used to handle them, it is imperative that the entire school know the importance of the effort on which it is embarked. Support for the project will not come from those who misunderstand it. The researchers have the difficult task of paring down their demands to those essential conditions which will govern the usefulness of the data, while maintaining the spirit of cooperation upon which the entire enterprise depends.

3
The Sample for School-Linked Evaluation

Defining the Sample Population

In any evaluation, a basic methodological decision relates to defining the population in which the program will be assessed; will only *recipients* of its services be included, or will effects be measured among all who are eligible for those services? When educational or clinical programs are evaluated by looking only at those who receive specific services, the effectiveness of the program's offerings is assessed by measuring change among those who are, in effect, its clients. We prefer to put school-linked initiatives to a harsher test. We measure the effects of a program on all of those who are eligible to use it. In that way, the study will measure the program's ability to *diffuse* knowledge and to *recruit* clients among its entire target population, rather than restricting the evaluation to the program's effects on the self-selected subset which presents for individual service.

Who comprises that "target"? Clearly, the base will be different when investigating the proportions of all students in the school who receive a given service from *service records*, as opposed to estimating the same proportion from the *aggregate survey data*. In the first case, the number eligible for the service includes all students in the school; in the second case, both the numerator and the denominator are drawn from the survey itself. Ideally, the two sources of information should not be mixed. For example, if the *number served* is drawn from the service records, and the *number eligible* is based on only the number of respondents to the survey, there will almost certainly be an overestimate of proportions served. It is the actual base number in the school which is needed in that proportion, and that is a surprisingly complicated number to develop. Although the number of students in the survey sample (those who completed the survey) is considerably smaller than the number in the school, the work we do in defining the school's entire population is useful in exploring the generalizability of the survey findings. It tells us who was available for study, and what happened to the school sample over time.

In a school program, on the simplest level, defining the eligible population appears easy: the denominator can simply represent all the students attending the school during a specific time period. It is, by definition, a closed population, more uniquely specified than a neighborhood or a community, a village or a city. This is a group of persons all of whom are eligible for the program's services and are (or should be) informed of its availability; they have prescribed and equal access to the program's staff and facilities.

Nonetheless, there are many problems associated with defining the sample in a school context. They can be divided into (1) problems that are common to all school settings; (2) problems that involve some local differences, often the kinds of historical changes to which we have alluded previously; and a category important enough to deal with separately; (3) problems of dropouts, absentees, and transfers. Although common to all schools, these issues have to be dealt with in the context of each school system, its record-keeping capacity, and its special types of schools.

Problems Common to All School Settings

In the first category are issues associated with movement into and out of schools due to (1) the normal flow of new students into all grades, (2) the passage of students through grade levels, and (3) the graduation of old students from junior and senior high schools.

Each year, large numbers of young people register for each specific school; they may or may not attend it, and some of them graduate, are promoted, or are transferred into other schools. There are also new students who enter throughout the school year. Thus, even without taking local idiosyncratic differences into account, researchers are dealing with transient, fluctuating populations. The obvious "authority" should be the registration rolls compiled by the school system, usually available as public access tapes. Under the Freedom of Information Act, these should be accessible on request. However, these rolls themselves are in constant flux, and are reissued in order to keep them current—sometimes monthly, sometimes weekly, and in some cases even daily. If a count is needed on which to base the denominator for an evaluation, one of these rolls needs to be selected. Although that choice is fairly arbitrary, it is often recommended that the November rolls be used, because there has been time for early errors in registration to be corrected, and because by waiting for a few months after the opening of the school year, one can best ensure that late registrants will be included. The November rolls may be looked on as maximal, because adjustments for dropouts are generally not made until later in the year.

Much more difficult is the determination of the numbers of individuals exposed in a school over a two- or three-year period. Some students continue, some leave, and some enter, so without tracking individuals, no accurate count of the number ever exposed to a multiyear program can be made. A rough estimate can be based on an enumeration of the numbers of new and old students each year. In that case, the total number equals the number of students the first year plus the numbers of new students added during the course of the first year and in subsequent years. Depending on the level of sophistication in a given school system's computer system, this information may or may not be easily available; some schools have the capacity to generate "running enrollment" data. They count total enrollment over a given period, starting with any entry date of choice, and adding all who enter over time. (This should not be confused with the net rolls discussed previously; they are "snapshots" of a given moment, whereas a running enrollment total describes all individuals ever enrolled in a school over time.) Note that this kind of estimate, whether calculated by the researchers on the basis of new students, or generated by the school system as a running enrollment, represents the total number *ever exposed* to a program in a school over a given time period, but says nothing of *how long each student continued to be exposed,* because it does not include information on how long each student remained in attendance at a program school. It adds those who enter but does not subtract those who leave.

Still other counts that can be used are the school's own attendance forms. Usually these can be obtained as homeroom lists, which, as we previously noted, are useful in packaging the questionnaires. Of course, the numbers of completed questionnaires are lower than the rolls because they do not include the day's absentees (nor refusals, should there be any). However, even the full homeroom rosters are likely to be lower than the school system's official rolls; chronic absentees and dropouts generally do not appear on homeroom lists, although they may remain on school rolls until officially terminated after the age of sixteen. In our evaluation, a rigorous test of program impact is applied to the program: when computing percentages served with a particular service, all registered students on any of the rolls are used for the school estimate, in order to include all possible participants. A simpler system, sufficient for most purposes, would utilize November rolls. Even then, the program may never have a chance to reach some of the students with any services at all.

It may be that even more specific information is required, so that the services to individuals in the school may be seen as a proportion of all individual exposures to the program. For example, if the question were asked: "How many student-months of exposure to the program were received by a student body of 1,500 a year, 500 of whom were new each year, over a three-year period?" the running enrollment alone might not be sufficient. In that case, withdrawals would need to be considered as well as additions, and the task becomes more difficult. The numbers of students leaving for graduation, and transferring in the course of the year and at the end of the year can be approximated with the help of the school, but calculating months of exposure to the program by grade or age demands more detail. In our case, a cost-effectiveness appraisal and our basic research requirements necessitated the inclusion of all students in the school in the data set. The school system provided tapes of all students in the schools at several times in each school year; all students were entered by name and student identification number so that total eligible student-months in the program schools could be estimated both in the aggregate and by individual. (Note the need to preserve confidentiality when names are in the records. In our program, all students attending the clinic signed consent for the use of their records for research; other students' records originally included only the public access information provided by the schools. When linked to services, names were removed and only numbers appear in the research files.) This exhaustive (and exhausting) process should only be undertaken if the research will justify the input of time and energy it requires.

Problems Specific to Individual School Settings

In the second category are issues related to changes in the composition of the schools, in the feeder schools from which students are drawn, and transfers between schools. There will, no doubt, be relatively small school systems in which all or most students of a given age are in a single middle, junior, or senior high, but in large urban centers that is far from true. In these school systems, there are frequently changes which need to be monitored if program effects are to be accurately assessed.

Things happen in the real world that are not allowed to happen in the laboratory, and real-world evaluation often has to "make do" with local idiosyncrasies that create far from ideal experimental conditions. It must not do so by ignoring these happenings, but by recognizing them and making specific adjustments to account for them. Evaluators should report these adjustments openly, so that others can judge whether or not the problem has been met and to what extent the findings are contaminated by a problem that will not go away. But adjustments are usually possible as long as the condition is known, and that requires close and intimate contact with the schools and school systems under investigation.

Many of these problems are created by what can be described as "historical change" in the research environment. A school may change from a junior to a middle school, a senior high school can add a ninth grade where previously it began in the tenth, new schools can open in an area, and feeder schools can change. In the first two cases, merely controlling the grades included in the comparison groups can handle the problem. In the last two cases, however, conscientious investigation into the effects of these changes is called for. It is possible, for example, that the feeder school can change without a serious alteration in the social, economic, and "risk" characteristics of the sample. Close consultation with those who know the community and those who know the schools can suggest whether this is the case; an examination of the aggregate characteristics provided by the school system can assist in making that determination. If there are indications that a real change has taken place, a much more serious problem exists. There is little that can be done to utilize the baseline data if a radical change in the composition of a school has taken place; fortunately, that possibility is extremely rare. After all, geographic locations in large urban communities rarely change in the short term, and schools are usually the offspring of a geographic environment. One might speculate that if such an event did take place, all might not be lost if new baseline data were collected when such a change went into effect. To all intents and purposes, those new data would be equivalent to baseline data, because so large a proportion of the young people would not yet have been exposed to the program. Much more likely are the kinds of changes that affect some limited subgroup within the school, and those can generally be handled by excluding aberrational subgroups from the analysis. Administering the survey to the entire school, being careful to include variables (for example, year transferred, school from which transferred), will still permit a great deal of accuracy in the comparison groups.

Another example of a totally local phenomenon, restricted in time and place to one administration of a survey, is the omission of one or more homerooms, classrooms, or subgroups from the day's survey recipients. Most commonly, this will be due to class trips or special events. Sometimes it can be more difficult to determine the effects of an omission, when only a subset of a grade is involved. Such an event occurred, unfortunately, in one round of the Hopkins study. A few homerooms of twelfth graders did not complete the third year's survey; when it was discovered that these homerooms selectively included the most highly motivated groups of seniors, it was determined that their omission would bias any comparison. Therefore, it was necessary to eliminate all twelfth graders from both the baseline and the follow-up data when comparisons involved that round of the survey. As this example suggests, the more specific the information available to the researchers, the more specific can be the adjustments, and thus the impact of the aberration on the evaluation can be minimized. It should be stressed, however, that the adjustment, however small, must be made if the final evaluation is to be credible. Without such an adjustment, it is quite possible that true program effects might be missed.

Dropouts, Absentees, and Transfers

All of the problems encountered in defining the population are complicated by dropouts, absentees, and transfers. Once students enter a school, they leave by one of four routes. They graduate (or in the case of middle and junior highs, are promoted to other schools in the system); they drop out or terminate their schooling in that school system; they transfer within the system; or they become chronic absentees who, by virtue of being younger than the legal age of termination and having gone through no formal termination procedure, are neither present nor officially on the termination rolls. (The last category is something of a catch-22: because the law states that students must stay in school until age sixteen, they can only be legally terminated for specified reasons, including, for example, transfer to another jurisdiction, institutionalization or ill health, and the school system's observation that they do not belong in school. The fourteen-year old student who simply stops attending school, without a termination interview, will often only appear as an absentee.)

It seems obvious that systematic changes in any of these "exit" routes could affect the evaluation. For example, if there were a significant decrease in the female dropout rate, it could be because many students who formerly had dropped out when pregnant remained in the school; in that case, the program would appear to have increased the pregnancy rate in the school when, indeed, it had merely been successful in meeting one of its auxiliary goals, encouraging pregnant girls to complete their education. Similarly, if an absentee rate falls, a program with a strong comprehensive health component might prove to have been particularly successful by reducing acute illness among its chronically ill; however, if it therefore retains more marginally healthy students, measures of certain health parameters might appear to increase. These relationships are complex and can never be completely sorted out, but basic assumptions and decisions with reference to those who leave the school need to be made.

Dropouts. Some proportion of the female students who drop out of school do so because they are pregnant; the exact numbers are rarely available but only certain dropout "codes" are likely places for them to appear on the school's termination rolls. Unfortunately, once a student has reached age sixteen, no code or reason for dropping out is required. Some subset of these young women are probably pregnant. Our study employed a method of handling the dropout dilemma, based on the following assumptions:

1. Although a program may affect dropout rates overall, there is little reason to believe that it will, in the short term, affect the proportion of all dropouts who do so because of a pregnancy.

2. If the overall dropout rate, in all the categories in which pregnant students might appear, changes systematically in the years immediately preceding, during, and immediately following the program, further exploration of dropouts will be necessary, especially if the systematic change is of a magnitude to affect overall rates.

3. If those rates remain constant, or continue to show small and random fluctuations during the program years as they did prior to and/or following the program, it can be assumed that they were not systematically affected. In that case, they can be ignored.

Material on those rates can be obtained from the school system, and should be checked for a number of years pre-program (and post-program if the intervention terminates) as well as during several program years. Clear definition of the assumptions and procedures used in the evaluation is essential to the credibility of the study since dropouts, transfers, and absentees may be crucial to the delineation of the sample.

Absentees. The same procedure can be applied to absentees. Clearly, a radical or systematic difference will have to be accounted for, but as long as the patterns look the same, it would be difficult to make a case for program effects, on the one hand, or contamination of the sample, on the other. Absentee information can be obtained for all students, or summary lists can be requested based on different numbers of days absent; the researchers can request lists of students absent 45 days a year or more, 100 days a year or more, and so on. A decision will have to be made as to what level will be treated not merely as an absentee but as a chronic absentee or a dropout, a decision which can be made in consultation with the school system. A decision will also have to be made about the inclusion of these students in the denominator. We used all the rolls, (and recommend using the entire November rolls) and did not subtract a number for chronic absenteeism. As explained previously, that decision puts a burden on the program, since its percent served will be minimized if students are included in the school roster whom the staff could not, with their best efforts, have reached.

Transfers. Some transfers appear on termination lists when families move to other jurisdictions or transfer their children to private or parochial schools. Numbers will generally be very small from individual schools; these transfers will probably be random, and therefore can be ignored for evaluation purposes. (One can conceive of times when that was not the case; the exodus of white students from Southern public schools at the time of school integration would be an extreme, nonrandom example. It is probably unlikely that an evaluator will find that kind of historical contamination in his or her particular sample, but the eventuality is not without possibility.)

Other types of transfers that could affect an evaluation were dealt with previously, when we discussed such historical changes as the redistricting of a school. As noted in the preceding, if a particular, numerically significant subgroup at greater or lesser risk is moved in or out en masse, there is little that can be done to retrieve the study; utilization of other subgroups who can be identified in the aggregate data may still be possible, but only if the analysis proceeds with extreme caution. This is an eventuality any researcher hopes will never occur.

Much more likely, and central to an evaluation, are *specific transfers for reasons related to the purposes of the program.* For example, if measuring delinquency, transfers to training schools obviously could not be ignored. Similarly, in a reproductive health program, transfers to schools maintained for pregnant teens must be counted, since they may well account for a significant proportion of the pregnancies in a given school. Fortunately, the cooperation of the school system can once again smooth the way. In the Hopkins program, lists were obtained of all transfers to the relevant school for three years before the program, during the program, and for a year following it. Dates of conception were calculated by subtracting nine months from the estimated date of confinement, which was a part of each girl's record. Schools of origin were listed, as were dates of transfer. Thus, the members of each grade in the study schools who, but for a pregnancy, would probably be in the aggregate data, were added to both numerators and denominators when pregnancy rates were calculated. We feel that the accuracy of our estimates of conception rates was greatly improved by including a subset all of whom, by the fact of their transfer, belonged in the numerator and significantly affected a crucial outcome measure.

It should be clear from the preceding paragraphs that describing a school population, counting its members, and defining its limitations is not quite as simple as it looks. Nonetheless, it is a great deal simpler than defining the sample in most community-based programs. Furthermore, there are several bonuses that come from working in a circumscribed setting, especially in an institutional setting that is recognized as an official entity, one that constantly counts its members, and one many of whose aggregate characteristics have already been described. School systems create and maintain large amounts of data. Some of them are available as public access data, and some can be run, when computerized systems permit, for the researcher who has taken the time to build trust. Absentee and dropout information, economic estimators (for example, percent free lunch), and educational estimators (for example, percent promoted, percent graduated, percent repeaters, grade averages) are all available as aggregate measures. These data can be useful in defining the characteristics of the sample, in choosing control schools, and finally in assessing the generalizability of the findings. Furthermore, this is a population in which the detail exists, down to an individual, name-identified level, should the researcher require it, whereas on the aggregate level, characteristics are known that might otherwise be difficult, time consuming, or perhaps impossible to collect.

It should also be clear that in defining the *whole school samples* we learn a good deal we need to know about how generalizable and how accurate the evaluation is likely to be, even though it is based on the smaller *survey sample*. We learn how similar the school populations are "before" and "after," who is included and who may be missing from the sample, whether there is any bias to the sample, and how similar the experimental and control schools are—all essential pieces of information when we evaluate the evaluation itself.

The Use and Limits of Controls

Anyone who has read the results of research, whether or not he or she has been involved in carrying it out, knows the importance of a comparison group. "Better than what?" "Lower than what?" are the questions we commonly ask when assessing the value of research findings. As discussed in chapter 1, social research in the real world requires that a number of compromises be made, since random assignment of equivalent populations to experimental and nonexperimental sites is rarely possible. In the case of school-based research, we have no control over who attends one school or another, and can only estimate on a few available parameters the equivalence of separate school populations.

The questions that must be answered, however, if the evaluation is to be of any value at all are, "How do we know that changes that occurred in the program schools are attributable to the program? How do we know they were not occurring all over the area at the same time?" These questions require the use of a control school, and the more equivalent that school is, the more certain we can be that the program was, indeed, the key to the observed *change*. Note that the emphasis here is on change. As suggested previously, it is change over time which is the outcome of interest, whatever particular effect is under study. This focus on change means that we are comparing changes that may have occurred in the program schools with changes that may have occurred in non-program schools during the same time period. We are *not* comparing the absolute level of a given variable in one school with its level in another, either at the beginning or the end of the time period. We are assessing the impact of the program in the experimental setting, and using the control population to assure ourselves that the effects we observe are not merely secular changes that were likely to affect all the young people in the jurisdiction, whether or not the intervention was in place.

We emphasize this point because it appears to be very difficult to find schools, even within the same school system, that are truly identical in all their relevant population characteristics. Schools differ in their geographic, economic, racial, and ethnic distributions; the proportions of their students who are male and female may differ, and their educational levels, rates of promotion and graduation, and dropout and repeat rates may differ as well. There may even be small differences in curriculum, with some special units incorporated by one principal, some special program incorporated by another. When populations differ, there is no reason to assume that the absolute values of relevant characteristics will be the same. It is not surprising that one population may report somewhat higher substance use and another a higher pregnancy rate, or even that one reports a higher abortion rate and another a higher rate of childbearing. These differences need not invalidate the use of the schools as controls for one another *if the focus of the study remains on relative change in variables of interest over time,* not on their absolute levels at any one period.

It should be stressed that, even while acknowledging the difficulty in matching schools, every effort needs to be made to match them as closely as possible. Controls should be selected from areas of the city (or other jurisdiction) as similar in economic level and social status to the experimental sites as possible. On some variables, equivalence can be augmented in the analysis phase; for example, if the racial or gender mix is somewhat different, race and sex subgroups can be matched in the final analysis. But samples that differ radically in a number of background characteristics make a poor match. There are controls that can be applied, however, to assure useful comparisons, when the basic requirements outlined here have been met: the collection of reliable baseline and follow-up data from basically equivalent study and control groups.

Rounds, Exposures, and Grade Levels

With membership in the sample defined, the model is based on the comparison of aggregate characteristics before and after exposure to the program. At first glance, it might appear that the assessment can be achieved with a separate comparison of Round I, administered before the program's onset, with Rounds II, III, and IV, administered at the end of school years one, two, and three, respectively. In fact, the movement of students in, out, and through the schools confounds the comparison unless stringent controls are applied to determine the exact exposure of each student in the aggregate population.

For our purposes, "exposure" is defined simply as presence in a school in which the program is in place. It is not to be confused with "utilization" of any particular component of the program. A student who has had no contact with the staff is considered "exposed" if the student is in a program school. Therefore, there is no element of self-selection in determining who is in the sample. This is important to the validity of the evaluation, since program assessments are often contaminated when only a self-selected group is available for study. In the Hopkins project, as in most service programs, those who actually utilized most services did so because they chose to. There was only one component of service that did not involve an element of self-selection; class lectures were heard by the vast majority of students whether or not they made any effort to seek out the program's staff. Even in the case of the class lectures, however, there was a higher probability that a frequent absentee would miss one than a student whose attendance was regular. Self-selection, then, would bias the comparison if only those *using* one or another service were compared; this would invalidate the concept of measuring the program's impact on an entire school population. The aggregate data from all students in the school makes for an unbiased sample.

We have said that a number based on the enumeration of all students on the November rolls can be used as the sample size when developing percentages of students served with group or individual services. The large subsample of those students actually present on the day of the survey is the population available for comparison when using the aggregate data. Within that sample, the questionnaire identifies the student's *present grade*, the *grade* in which the student *entered* the program school, and the *school* from which the student came. Exposure is defined as the number of school years in a program school, calculated from these three variables. The comparisons of interest, then, are between the entire sample at first administration, (figure 1–1) and those surveyed at later periods who were exposed for one, two or three years.

Exposure varies first of all by grade and by individual. Students in certain grades can have an exposure of only one year, whenever a program begins, because the program starts at their current grade level. Other students can only have two years' exposure because the program begins one grade below their present grade level. Next, exposure varies by round. If a round is administered in spring of the first year, all the students who take it are exposed for one year. Exposures of two or three years, however, involve only subsets of the sample. Finally, exposure varies by school. In the current case, seventh graders in the junior high and ninth graders in the senior high can only be exposed for one year, even if the program has been in place for many years; ninth graders in the junior high school in the last year of the program, however, could have been exposed for one, two, or three years. Thus, exposures are related not only to *grade* and *round*, but to *school*, with those who move from a program junior high to a program senior high having the potential for a longer exposure than those who transfer in from other, non-program settings.

Exposure also varies by individual, since an individual student can have entered in the year a follow-up survey is administered, or can have been present in the school from the time the program was put in place. The survey variables allow us to identify the student who has been exposed for a shorter period than the majority of his or her classmates. No adjustment is made for fractions of the school year; the number of students entering during the year is small relative to the entire student body, and the data would be difficult to collect and even more cumbersome to utilize. Figure 3–1 shows the relationships between grade, school, round, and exposure; this format can be adapted to other programs' timetables, once the principles on which it is based are understood. Note that not only exposure and round are shown separately, but grade. As the previous paragraphs indicate, exposure varies by grade. Furthermore, there are substantive reasons to control by grade, as well as methodological reasons. In a population whose characteristics are as age dependent as they are in adolescence, age controls are important. In this

		Junior High School			Senior High School				
Round	Exposure	7	8	9a	9b	10a	10b	11	12
I	0								
II + subset of III and IV	1								
III + subset of IV	2	✕			✕				
IV	3	✕	✕		✕		✕		

OR

III + IV	≥ 2	✕			✕				

Note: 9a is the ninth grade in the junior high school; 9b the ninth grade in the senior high school. 10a is the subset of the tenth grade consisting of students who entered the senior high from the program junior high school; 10b consists of all other tenth graders.

Figure 3–1. Relationship of Rounds, Grades, and Exposures

model, individual grades become a proxy for age, and comparisons aggregated by grade will form the basis of the analytic model.

In chapter 5, when we discuss details of the analytic methodology, we will address particular problems which must be addressed in comparing across exposures. What needs to be stressed here, however, is the importance of using exposures rather than rounds. When rounds are compared, they are seriously contaminated by the limitations we have just described, and the results they will give, when a round is used as a "stand-in" for exposure, will simply be incorrect. Although the simplicity of such a comparison is tempting, it will not yield a satisfactory evaluation of the program's true effects.

Minimal Requirements for Defining the Sample

The methods described in this chapter may be more detailed and more complex than many evaluators wish to attempt. What, at a minimum, is necessary in a simplified evaluation—one to be used not for basic research or replication, but as a tool for the providers themselves?

First, a basic number will be needed to serve as the denominator in measuring the percentage reached with any given service. A simple count of male and female students, obtained from the principal, is probably enough; it is preferable to choose a midpoint in the year for this estimate. Even an old-fashioned card file to keep track of all students, and their service records, could be enough. On the other hand, when it comes to survey data, the denominator will be the number of respondents. This number, plus the numbers of refusals and absentees the school reports, can serve as an estimate of the number of students eligible for service.

Second, a report can be obtained from the school system on certain aggregate characteristics identified at a single point in time. A comparison of these reports across several years can be used to assure the evaluators that there are no substantive and/or systematic changes in the populations with which they are dealing. Variables of interest could include dropout rates, absentee rates, promotion and repeater rates, mean grade averages, percentages receiving free and partially paid lunches. Only if comparisons show significant differences in any of these parameters will the composition of the student body need to be examined in the detail previously described. Third, similar aggregate reports can be obtained to help in the selection of control schools.

Unfortunately, as stressed in the last section, the analytic methodology for comparing over exposures and grades cannot be similarly simplified. Once figure 3–1 is understood, a similar chart can be drawn, indicating which exposure/grade/round categories will be useful in performing the final evaluation. If the appropriate questions are asked in the survey instrument, a simple computer program can be used to assign correct exposure subgroups. We cannot emphasize too strongly the importance of using these "exposure" controls, since comparison across rounds, in the absence of any information on exposure, might yield a very negative evaluation of a program that has, indeed, been extremely successful.

4
The Survey Instrument

Since the basic data collection tool for the program evaluation is a student self-administered questionnaire, the structure of that instrument is of utmost importance. It will necessarily involve some degree of compromise, not only for purposes of parsimony but because the subject matter is often sensitive. Some will maintain that the importance of information in each area of investigation must be weighed against the reactions of the public to the nature of the questions. Ultimately, one would hope that decisions would be made on the scientific basis of "the need to know." When the logic of the questionnaire is explained, there is often a gratifying level of acceptance of even the most personal of explorations. The actual questionnaires presented in appendix C are the final questionnaires used at the end of the program in the program schools and, with adjustments we shall describe, in the non-program schools. It should be recalled that the purpose of the questionnaire is to collect the same information at several points in time, in order to do longitudinal analysis on an aggregate basis. This permits the researchers to assess program outcome measures, and also allows an opportunity for basic research, which may focus on change over time but is more likely to utilize data collected prior to, or in the absence of, program.

The basic content remained the same for the several rounds described in chapter 1, although there were some changes in content and actual questions, which will be discussed. When such changes were made, care had to be taken in their instrumentation in order to remain consistent in the measurement of major outcome variables. Although one often learns to assess a characteristic with greater accuracy in the course of a study such as ours, changes in measurement instruments must be made with extreme caution if pre- and post-test results are to be truly comparable. The instruments which appear in appendix C are those that were used in the program schools; questions that ask the students directly about the program itself do not appear when the questionnaire is administered in the control sites.

There were six questionnaire types, numbered, for researchers' convenience, 1 through 6. Types 1 and 2 were given to ninth- through twelfth-grade males, types 3 and 4 to ninth- through twelfth-grade females. (These four types are included as appendix C.) Types 5 and 6, given to males and females, respectively, were the seventh- and eighth-grade versions. (In this chapter, the term *older students* will refer to students given questionnaire types 1 through 4 and *younger students* will refer to those given questionnaire types 5 and 6.) Colors were useful to distinguish the questionnaire types, especially to enable teachers to give males and females in the same classroom the correct questionnaires.

In any study, there are more questions researchers want to ask than time in which to ask them. A split sample can therefore be used to ask some questions of only one-half of the respondents; these should be questions that require a smaller sample, are of secondary importance, or parallel other questions asked of the entire population. In the present study, this method was used for the ninth- through twelfth-grade students. A limited number of questions were designated for this purpose; hence there are two questionnaire types for each sex, each identified with a different number. An even number of questionnaires of each type were distributed to each sex in each class so that answers to most questions would be available from all students, and answers to a small set of questions from one-half of the students. As the questionnaires are described in the following pages, it should be noted that the split sample questions are not crucial to the behavioral outcome measures being evaluated. They may be behavioral, attitudinal, or informational, but are generally questions that are reasonably unambiguous to code, or, in some cases, they are exploratory in nature.

Still other differences separated the questionnaires given younger students; questionnaire types 5 and 6 were simpler and shorter than the instruments administered to older students. The decision not to use a split sample for younger respondents is based, in the current study, on the need for a shorter instrument and on numbers: fewer students were available. A split sample should not be considered unless one-half of the students in the relevant grades constitute a sufficiently large sample for the variables under study.

The questions on program use are the same on all questionnaires administered to the program schools. The same basic questionnaires were used in the control schools, with the exception of the items dealing with program use. As described in figure 1–1, the questionnaires were administered at $time_1$ and $time_4$ in all four schools, and in the program schools at two intervening periods. An example of a "historical" change intervening during the time period of the study was evidenced in the present project: between $time_1$ and $time_4$, the grade composition of the non-program junior high school had changed; it had become a middle school, consisting of grades six through eight instead of grades seven through nine. The senior high school consisted of grades nine through twelve, so the ninth grade continued to be available. This potential problem was solved by administering the same questionnaires to the sixth through eighth graders, but omitting the sixth graders' data from the evaluation in order that the populations remain thoroughly comparable. This local example is cited to focus attention on the need to maintain close contact with the school systems under scrutiny. When administering an evaluation tool to populations not well known to the researchers, it is all too easy to miss changes that do not appear important to those less familiar with the stringent demands of research protocols. As we suggested in chapter 3, there are generally ways of compensating for such changes, but only if one knows that the potential problem exists.

Although the pages that follow will describe the instrument used in the index program in some detail, some evaluators may not wish to ask questions in precisely these ways, nor to structure their questionnaires similarly. Many of these questions, however, have been carefully honed, utilizing the experience of many researchers who have explored these topics in adolescent populations, beginning with the Zelnik/Kantner National Survey of Young Women in 1971. When there are known pitfalls which must be avoided in the rephrasing of important variables, we will indicate why the phrases used are of particular importance. It may be that evaluators will want a trimmed, streamlined version of these questionnaires; when the objective is program assessment only, and no basic research is anticipated, a briefer version may be appropriate. We will specify at the end of the chapter those variables that are essential even to the most focused evaluation. Other researchers will wish to expand this format to include variables specific to their program offerings. For example, our cursory treatment of substance use will need to be expanded in some settings, to include history, more specification of substance types, and other aspects of use that need exploration. Similarly, comprehensive health programs will, no doubt, add many questions on sources of health care, utilization of health services, nutrition, and a wide range of other health-related topics. Expansion of this type will require that the number of questions focused on sexuality, contraception, and fertility be limited, however important pregnancy reduction is to the program at hand. Nonetheless, since these are frequently among the most sensitive questions, the following detailed discussion should be of interest.

Questionnaire construction is an exacting discipline. Knowing decisions made during the study, and the reasons for those decisions, may help future researchers in the design process. Furthermore, if use of similar formats were to permit comparison between many individual data sets, a real contribution could be made to the field of adolescent research.

Constructing the Survey Instrument

Background/Demographic Variables

The questionnaire begins with several background/demographic items to be used for both evaluation and basic research. These are necessary in order to describe the student population and to enable researchers to examine differences among subgroups of students. Items include age, date of birth, present grade, grade average, race, marital status, religion, religiosity, foster care history, and aspired education. Whether or not a student is Hispanic should be asked as a question separate from that on race, since both black and white students may be of Hispanic background.

By asking the grade in which respondents entered the school, the school from which they came, and their present grade, it is possible to assess each student's length of exposure to the program (see chapter 3). It could be more appropriate to explore the *years* a student has been in the school, rather than the *grade* in which the student entered, because of the relatively high rate of repeaters in many of the nation's schools (especially true in the junior high schools in the current program). However, the student can probably give a more accurate response to the question as asked herein; a follow-up question "Did you repeat any grades since you came to this school?" would permit even more specific assessment of exposure.

The preceding information was asked on every questionnaire in every round in the Hopkins study, with only a few minor modifications in the questions or the responses allowed. The questions are well tested and appear to yield valid responses. Only one question, that on aspired education, was asked in different forms. In Rounds I and II, respondents were asked to circle the highest year of school or college they thought they would complete; they were also asked whether they expected to take job training or to enter military service. In Rounds III and IV, they were asked if they expected to get more education after finishing school, what their educational plans were if they expected to get more, and, again, whether they planned to enter military service. The change in the question was made because there are some ways to continue an education that are not necessarily related to grade level (for example, GED [the alternative diploma for those tested outside the school setting]), and because expectations, although still hypothetical, are not as vague as the original phrasing allowed.

It may be important, albeit for basic research only, to know who among the students has siblings in the same school or in another school being assessed by the same questionnaire. This could influence analysis if one wishes to ensure independent samples on variables that involve parent information. For example, if one examines maternal characteristics, and a mother has two children in the school, she would be included twice. This would violate some of the assumptions of independence which are made when using statistical methodology. In some rounds, a question on sibling information asked students whether they had siblings attending the same school that they attended. However, matching siblings requires detailed information not available in these anonymous questionnaires; therefore, the final question asks only how many older and younger brothers and older and younger sisters the respondent has, and does not permit analysis of independent family units.

Other background questions are scattered throughout the questionnaire. In order to compute the mother's age at her first birth, ages of the respondent's mother and of the mother's oldest child are requested. Each older boy is asked questions about his father as well, including age, age of his oldest child, whether he lives in the household, how often the respondent sees his father, and with whom he is more likely to talk over a problem—his mother or father. These respondents are also asked whether they have held a job for which they received pay. Although this information on male parenthood and on job history would have been interesting whether the respondent was male or female, the demands of the fertility history in female questionnaires made it impossible to include as many background questions. Since the entire questionnaire should be restricted to less than an hour (normally one school period), many qustions need to be pared from the final instrument; however, the opportunity to get information such as this, even if only from male students, is worth taking.

One-half of the ninth- through twelfth-grade respondents (a split sample) and all of the younger respondents are asked to describe who presently lives in their households, whether they have ever had sex education courses, where they have had them and their contents, and what was the highest grade of school completed by their mothers.

Some new background/demographic variables were introduced in the final questionnaire included in appendix C. Older students are asked five yes/no questions about sources of household income and government subsidized services in order to get some measure of socioeconomic status. These questions deal with aspects of the families' financial status which many experts suggest are well known by the young people involved. Attempts to identify socioeconomic status among teenagers are not successful if income is used as a measure; they rarely have that information. In the final version, they are also asked whether they had a job during the previous summer for pay, and if so, they are asked in an open-ended question what that job was.

In an attempt to determine maturation status for males, all males are asked if they have had their first wet dream yet; in the later rounds of this study, the question is phrased to ask whether they have ever "come," with *wet dream* used as a parenthetical term of definition. This was done after research had shown that for this population, the events occurred at the same age whether as intercourse or nocturnal emission. The questions can be separated for use with other populations. All females are asked if they have "come on yet," again with "first monthly period" as a parenthetical definition. All respondents are then asked when the first such event took place, and how old they were at the time. This area of inquiry can be used as an example of a pervasive issue in survey design: the need to use terminology the young people understand, without falling into a level of slang or street language that is particularly offensive to some readers. Intimate involvement with providers who know and work with similar groups of teenagers is a distinct advantage. "Come on," in this case, is a very local idiom, one not appropriate to other areas of the country. Only those who know the subjects well can give this guidance. If no reliable source is available for the appropriate idiom, focus groups with parallel populations are useful. Care must be taken *not* to use individuals who may eventually be included in the study population.

In rounds of survey administration after the first, all program respondents are asked if they have taken the questionnaire before; after the second round, they can be asked how many times they have done so.

All respondents are asked where they learned most about sex and birth control. If the researchers seek only *one* answer, the question must emphasize "the *one* place" where most was learned; without that specification, respondents tend to check more than one answer. In this and other questions, the determination should be made in advance by the survey designers as to whether multiple answers or a single choice is permitted, and the question must be phrased accordingly.

In an attempt to understand the adolescents' perceptions of their parents' attitudes, all questionnaire rounds have a series of questions asking respondents whether their parents would like it or not if they did not graduate from high school, had sex with their boyfriends/girlfriends, or became pregnant (or made a girl pregnant) while in school. In addition, students are asked whether, in the event of a pregnancy, their parents would want the pregnancy to result in a baby or an abortion. This appeared to be a more interesting question than an earlier version asking parents' feelings on abortion only, since it more clearly contrasts feelings about the two pregnancy outcomes. It should be recognized that questions such as these yield extremely "soft data." In this case, the young person is being asked to express a perception of another's perceptions, making it difficult to know how to use the information. It is an area which, nonetheless, seemed important to probe, because it reflects the family ambience in which the young person carries out his or her behavior. It can be argued that a parent's actual feelings may be less important than his or her offspring's perceptions of those feelings. Responses to questions such as these should be cautiously utilized in the analysis.

Although most researchers ask all students some basic question on ethnicity, more detailed background information may be of interest. In some schools, students come from many different ethnic or national backgrounds; this may be useful data for basic research. In the present study, students in the last round in the non-program schools were asked, in an open-ended question, to indicate the ethnic groups with which their parents identified, if any. Results suggest that this can yield interesting information, but responses cover so many nationalities in an ethnic white population that a judicious grouping of the responses is necessary before analysis can usefully be carried out. Unless numbers of students are large, and ethnic diversity a feature of the population, this question should probably be excluded from the instrument.

Knowledge Variables

In a program based, in any significant degree, on educational interventions, it is reasonable to believe that changes in the level of relevant knowledge might be observed. In fact, information may be all that education can change; there is little support for the notion that, *by itself,* it can change much else. Since the Hopkins project was in large measure an educational program, knowledge was one of the three outcome areas originally proposed as the basis for evaluation. The level of knowledge was expected to increase, and it did.

Questions in the survey should tap as many dimensions of relevant knowledge as possible, whatever the program, given the obvious time constraints. In any area of exploration, but especially in sensitive areas (sex, drugs, delinquency, and so on), care should be taken that informational questions be clearly informational; that is, that no element of "opinion" should confound them.

All ninth- through twelfth-grade students are asked seven true/false questions about the safety, use, and benefits of specific contraceptive methods, two questions about the risk of pregnancy, and one question about abortion. An index created from these ten questions becomes a summary measure, and is used to assess changes in sexual/contraceptive knowledge. The questions can, of course, be used individually, but the index probably gives a more realistic estimate.

Another informational question asks the respondents to check the time of the month during which a girl is most likely to get pregnant. A similar question has been used by other researchers; we differ, however, in our interpretation of the response. We allow for *two* correct answers, both of which can be interpreted as conducive to "protective" behavior, and therefore correct: "About two weeks after her period begins" and "Any time during the month." The latter is, indeed, what most sex education programs teach, and is especially appropriate among adolescents, whose cycles are frequently irregular. (In fact, this may be the reason researchers have found that so few teenagers appear to give the fourteen-day response; that is rarely what they have been taught.) The question is asked of all young students and one-half of the older students. The same respondents are asked four questions about the necessity of parents' permission for a teen to get reproductive health services. Younger students are asked if they have heard of syphilis, gonorrhea, and herpes.

It was suggested previously that *informational* questions should not be confused with *opinion* questions; if there is no correct answer, the subject is not an appropriate measure of knowledge. One question in the instrument described here appears to violate that commandment: it asks all students whether they have heard of eight nonpermanent contraceptive methods (including douche). If so, they are asked to rate each one as a very good, good, fair, or a poor way to keep a girl from getting pregnant. This question has become known as the "perception of method efficacy." It must be treated, as a whole, as "perception," but within judicious limits it can also be used to assess knowledge. Only extremes can be so used, if they are well accepted and documented as fact. For example, those who said withdrawal, rhythm, or douche are good or very good methods of preventing pregnancy were considered "wrong" (rhythm is included among these because, in an adolescent population that is uncertain of the timing of ovulation, and among whom a high proportion of irregular cycles makes the method extremely risky, it must be so considered.) Changes over time were examined in those percentages. However, when measuring the relevance of their perceptions of method efficacy to contraceptive use, for example, the responses are seen as attitudinal, which legitimately they are.

Older students are asked two series of questions, one about what they thought or did *before* they had ever had sex (if they have ever had sex) and a second about *now*. These questions were the following: whether sex could make a girl pregnant; whether the respondent would have a good chance of getting pregnant (or getting a girl pregnant) if she or he had sex; if the respondent had ever thought of getting birth control/condoms; if the respondent had ever talked to his or her partner about the risk of pregnancy and about birth control. The younger students are asked only one set of these questions without specifying the period of reference. This is clearly a mixed question, combining knowledge, attitudes, and behavior, and its component parts can be used either independently or relative one to the other. Only the first portion of the question, whether sex can make a girl pregnant, can be interpreted as reflective of the level of the respondent's knowledge.

Attitude Variables

Attitudes were from the outset another outcome area of interest. The program staff stressed "values" and sought to focus attention on the perceptions their students had of themselves and their personal behaviors. It was believed that attitudes might change, and since perceptions are difficult to tap, there were many more questions reflective of attitude than were used to assess knowledge. Overall, attitudes showed much less change than knowledge during the course of the program. Some of this is due to the fact that the students appeared to hold fairly responsible attitudes toward sex, contraception, pregnancy, and parenting before the program began and therefore there was less room for change. Researchers will want to make judicious choices in this area, because attitudinal data are always hard to interpret and, as tempting as this field is to explore, experience suggests that they tell us rather less about behavior than one might wish.

One type of question unique to this instrument asks the "best" ages for four different events to occur for a woman and for a man (for some events the words girl and boy are used instead). The events are the following: having sex for the first time, getting married, having a first baby (or becoming a father), and starting to date (this question is asked of younger students only). These four questions should not be asked consecutively; they should be widely scattered in the survey instrument, since the purpose is to obtain independent ages for the four events. Analyzing the responses independently and in juxtaposition will yield interesting insights.

Three other attitudinal questions are asked of all students, one each relating to sex, contraception, and pregnancy. All students are asked to check, on a continuum, the relationships in which it is "okay" for a boy and girl to have sex. They are asked whose responsibility it is to see that a girl does not get pregnant when having sex and for whom it is a problem to have a baby when one or both parents are in high school.

Many attitudinal questions are asked of each of the ninth- through twelfth-grade split samples, and many of these are asked of the younger students as well. One subset is asked attitudes related only to pregnancy and parenting. These questions include the following: whether these students think they could get pregnant (or get a girl pregnant) easily if they had sex; what a girl who got pregnant by a boy she does not love should do about the pregnancy; what their mothers would think and how they themselves would feel if they got pregnant (or got a girl pregnant); whether pregnancy is a good way to show you are an adult or to gain respect; whether children born to teens have more problems than those born to older parents; their desired number of children; whether they want to get married; reasons why becoming a mother or father now would be a problem; and under what circumstances it is all right for a woman to have an abortion.

The other subgroup is asked a series of true/false questions related to parental communication about sex, whether premarital sex is wrong, their partners' communication about and attitudes toward contraception, barriers to the use of contraception, whether they would only have sex if contraception was being used, and whether they would like to have a baby while in high school.

In order to assess more precisely the spectrum of opinion, a specific question is included on all versions asking whether it is important to be married before having a baby. Critics who disapprove of questionnaires of this type often suggest that questions about sexual behavior carry the implication that it is condoned. Survey instruments should include some questions which allow those who disapprove strongly of premarital sex, premarital conception, the use of contraception, and so on, to make their views known.

The split sample is used quite heavily for these questions, because they are less crucial to the evaluation. In fact, as indicated previously, in the index study they did not suggest the need for, nor the presence of, a great deal of change. This should not imply that as a programmatic focus they are unimportant. It may be that discussions of these concepts by the staff contributed to the students' ability to turn their responsible attitudes into behavior. In turn, the knowledge that their clients hold fairly responsible attitudes, whatever their conduct may be, can be helpful to the professionals who are working in this difficult field. We discuss this substantive area in some detail here because it is an example of the importance of cautious and sensitive interpretation: a set of variables should not be overinterpreted in the abstract but integrated into our understanding of the program strategy as a whole. Nonetheless, under the time constraints imposed on school questionnaires, especially those in comprehensive program settings with many areas to explore, the number of attitudinal variables can be reduced in future survey instruments without limiting their value.

Behavioral Variables

Of the three major outcome areas, knowledge, attitudes, and behavior, the last is clearly the most important. When programs include educational and clinical service components, one might expect to see positive changes in such behavioral areas as sexual onset, clinic use, contraceptive use, and pregnancy. These were all assessed in the Hopkins study, and all show changes in the direction of more responsible sexual conduct. The format of the questions, and their content, will be discussed here, and chapter 5 will address some of the analytic techniques which need to be utilized in understanding these complex variables. It should be noted that the nature of the information one seeks to collect on sexual behavior, especially in a program that focuses on reproductive health, is such as to require large numbers of individual questions. This is true for several reasons: (1) Although often combined under the rubric of "sexual behavior," the information we are seeking actually concerns several different areas—the sexual behavior itself, clinic behavior, contraceptive behavior, and fertility history. (2) There are issues of vocabulary involved, and questions frequently need to be phrased in several ways in order to be certain that the question the student is answering is, indeed, the one the researchers meant to ask. (3) We are often seeking to understand an entire history, not a single event; and (4) when looking at a history, it is important to establish the timing of these behaviors, relative not only to chronological age, but to one another. We will comment upon each of these issues in the following discussion.

All ninth- through twelfth-grade female respondents (whether or not they have been sexually active) are asked if they have ever been to a clinic or doctor to get birth control. If they have, they are asked detailed questions about their first visit: when it occurred, their age at that occurrence, where and why they went, the contraceptive method they received at that visit, how long they used the method received, and, if they stopped using it, why. (The last question provided little useful material.) They are also asked if they are presently using birth control pills.

All other groups are asked if they have ever been to a birth control clinic and, if so, younger females are asked what method they received and how long it was used. Boys are asked if they went with their girlfriends. In the final round, when effects of the program are being assessed, program school students are asked if the first birth control clinic they ever attended was the one attached to the Hopkins project.

Older male respondents are asked if they have ever obtained condoms from various listed sources and, if yes, when that first occurred and how old they were at the time. Younger males are simply asked if they have ever bought condoms.

The analysis can extend beyond the issue of whether or not respondents have *ever* been to a clinic; it can probe when, in relation to first having intercourse, that visit occurred. The timing of a clinic visit relative to first coitus is a useful variable when exploring females' exposure to pregnancy over time. Getting students to attend a clinic more promptly after sexual initiation, or, better, before that event, was therefore one of the goals of the program. In order to understand the delay that often occurs in reaching a professional facility, older girls were given a list of potential reasons for delay and asked to check those that made it hard for them to get birth control methods from a clinic. These questions have been well tested in prior research, and contribute to our understanding of the population. They can be adapted, adding potential reasons to the list that reflect local situations these may not cover. A similar approach can also be used to other types of services, as can the previous questions on the timing of service utilization. Whatever problem the intervention addresses, it is likely that timing is of importance, and barriers to prompt, professional assistance should be explored in a needs assessment or in an evaluation instrument.

All respondents are asked if they have ever had sexual intercourse. For those who have, information is collected about four facets of intercourse: the first event, the last event, coital frequency, and the number of partners with whom intercourse has occurred. Respondents are asked how old they were at their first experience, how old their partners were, and in what month and year that first sexual contact occurred. This event appears to be well recalled. It is an important variable, and the dating of the event relative to chronological age, schooling, contraception, conception, age of maturation, and so on, is of substantive interest. It needs definition in its local idiom as well as in formal English, and, as will be detailed here, it is a complicated variable to use. In one round, an added question attempted to ascertain, from females, the age at which they first had sex with a boy who was old enough to "come," and from the males, the age at which they first had sex when they were old enough to "come." This is a basic research issue, explored here because many respondents in the first round had cited a prepubertal age (premenarche for girls, pre-wet dream for boys) as their age of first intercourse. This raised some questions about the vocabulary of sexual onset: Can adolescents distinguish between prepubertal and postpubertal activity? How far apart, in age, are their responses to the two differently phrased questions? Should one ask the question in one way or the other, and what is the meaning of the response? Based on findings of this study, it still appears useful to ask the question as it appears in appendix C, with the understanding that the answers should be interpreted with some caution. They certainly give an estimate of early versus later coital activity. For the small number of females who place the events at two separate dates, there is no reason not to believe that event to have been prepubertal. For males, in permissive settings, nocturnal emissions and coital activity may simply be different expressions of the same developmental timetable; it may not be surprising that for almost equal numbers, one or the other comes first. Overall, even if the dates of first coitus sometimes reflect prepubertal behavior, they appear to be closely related to the age of puberty itself. When a question can be asked in a straightforward manner, as it appears in the basic questionnaire in appendix C, that is highly preferable. The auxiliary question, added in only one round, is phrased in a vernacular some critics might well find objectionable; unless there were an important reason to ask the question in this complex and colloquial way, we would always suggest going with the simpler, initial phrasing.

Only questionnaires for older respondents contain questions about last intercourse, coital frequency, and partners. Respondents are asked when they last had sex, how old they and their partners were, and their relationships at the time with their last sexual partners. When respondents were asked in earlier versions of the questionnaire how many times they had had sex in the last month, it was not clear what "last month" meant to the respondent; it could have been October, for example, if the survey was administered any time in November, or it could have been the thirty or thirty-one days immediately preceding the date of administration. Therefore, in the interest of accuracy, "last month" is redefined as "in the last four weeks" in the final version. The question "What is the *most* times you ever had sex in one month?" is not equivocal; *any* one-month period is implied. Because not everyone has sex with a person he or she would describe as a "girlfriend" or "boyfriend", the terms *girl* and *boy* are used in asking respondents how many partners they have ever had. These are a few examples of the precision required in the phrasing of questions if ambiguity is to be avoided in the coding and interpretation phases of the study.

Questions about contraceptive use are of major importance to evaluation. As will be discussed in detail in chapter 5, pregnancy rates require time to change. If program staff are in need of a quick assessment of impact, in one or two years time, for example, they cannot be given the information they seek from pregnancy rates. However, changes in clinic attendance or contraceptive use can signal the beginning of behavioral change, and the absence of such improvement can signal the need for programmatic review. For that reason, these complex variables require careful attention, as important behaviors in their own right, as markers for longer term change, and as indicators of the ways in which a program might be working to effect ultimate changes in fertility. Similarly, attendance at a substance use clinic, enrollment in a program, compliance with a regime, might signal program effects before one could document long-term, significant changes in substance use. Furthermore, as measures of program utilization, they are valuable variables in themselves.

The series of questions on contraceptive use begins with "ever use": if the respondent has ever used a contraceptive method, she or he is asked whether a method was used the first time she or he had sex, and how often the respondent has done something to keep herself (or to keep a girl) from getting pregnant since first method use. Then respondents are asked to check all the methods they or their partners have ever used. All respondents are asked to check the methods of birth control they or their partners used the last time they had intercourse; the list is large and includes "no method" as one choice.

In the interest of economy, it may be necessary to make choices between questions on "ever" use, "first" use, and "last" use; they give very different information. Experience with the variable *ever use* suggests that it tells very little about the habits of the respondent, and shows little correlation with any other variables reflecting protective behavior. It may, if answered in the affirmative, merely mean that the respondent has had several partners, and one, at one time, used some method, with or without the respondent being involved in that decision. It may, therefore, be related to long exposure and, in turn, to early sexual onset, which we know to be related to worse, not better, contraceptive practice. Conversely, it may be related to consistent, effective use. One might ask why it should be asked at all. Mainly, as a lead-in to the other questions; if the answer is "no, never," a skip pattern can carry respondents over other questions on contraception, or if no skip pattern is used, it can be useful in the data cleaning process (see the section on Data Preparation) to check on the reliability of the several responses.

On the other hand, use at last intercourse appears to be a good variable, and provides an estimate of the regularity of method use. Obviously, it is only an estimate, because even fairly reliable users might have missed on a single, random occasion. However, since it is a random occasion, it provides a useful estimate and in many studies has been shown to correlate well with other related attitudes and behaviors. Furthermore, it is generally a rather recent estimate; even if it has been a long time between last intercourse and administration of the survey, it is necessarily more recent than any other similar event. Especially if the date of that last event is known, it provides interesting insights in relation to other dated occurrences, such as clinic visit, utilization of the program facilities, age, and the like.

Another attempt was made to elicit some information about contraceptive history, and in particular on regularity of method use. Older students are asked whether they or their partners used a method at first coitus, and then are asked, "Since you first did anything to keep from getting pregnant, have you done something: always, most of the time, not very much, never." If this series is cited as an accurate measure of contraceptive history, it is probably not very useful. However, we interpret the response more as an attitude toward recent method use, and in combination with other variables, it yields additional insights. In view of the fact that many of the respondents have had histories of coital exposure covering many years, it is probably impossible in a single question on regularity of use to obtain a true historical measure. Therefore, the format recommended in appendix C comes as close to a summary description as possible, without requiring the detail that can only be elicited in a long and personal discussion of sexual and contraceptive history.

In some surveys, the question on regularity of use is simplified to "Have you used contraception: never, sometimes, always," or some variation of that format. The main problem with such a phraseology is that the "sometimes" category is too broad to be meaningful. It can apply to the young person who failed to use during the first month of coitus, then began to use and has used consistently ever since, to the irregular but fairly consistent user, and to the casual, occasional user. A little more accurate is the variation that includes "always, always since first use, sometimes, never." The version in the current questionnaire is the refinement we found useful; of course, all such questions contain compromises, made in the interest of brevity.

The final major outcome in behavior, the one that is bound to be cited as the measure of program success or failure, is pregnancy. The series of questions used to measure this dimension is different for older males and females, and also different for older and younger students. Older males are first asked whether they have ever had a "pregnancy scare" and how many times that has occurred. They are then asked if they have ever made a girl pregnant and, if so, how many times, how many times each outcome occurred, and how many different girls they have impregnated. They are also asked specific questions about the *last* pregnancy outcome, (or the current pregnancy): when they last made a girl pregnant, what its outcome was, and what contraceptive method they used at that conception, if any. Note that they are given a choice to establish whether they *know* the outcome; a forced choice, without "don't know," might encourage them to mask their ignorance. In addition, boys are asked to indicate whether or not they had wanted to get a girl pregnant so people would think "you're a man," and whether they or their partners had wanted the pregnancy before it occurred. Finally, they are asked about future plans for the pregnancy, if the girlfriend is currently pregnant. It is very hard to evaluate how good this series is, since there is really no external data with which it can be compared. The internal consistency is not as strong as one would hope, but the need for information on the male side of the pregnancy equation appears to be sufficiently strong, and the current dearth of information sufficiently serious, so that we would support any creative effort to acquire that understanding even if the data are known to be "soft."

The ninth- through twelfth-grade females are also asked whether they have ever experienced a pregnancy scare, and if so, how many times. We then move on to a series of questions designed to assess female pregnancy history. Although this is an area in which more reliable and valid data are available than can be elicited from males, it is still a difficult area to explore, and even more crucial to the study. Vocabulary, skip patterns, timing of the events, all complicate this series, which takes the final form shown in appendix C. Following it closely while reading this discussion will make the issues clearer.

These females are asked whether they have had any of four possible pregnancy outcomes, birth, miscarriage, abortion, or currently pregnant, each requiring a separate response. They are then asked how many of each outcome they have experienced. The third question in the pregnancy history asks what they did the *first* time they were pregnant. The respondent answers by filling in the date of outcome on the correct line for their first outcome, or the number of months pregnant if currently pregnant. The fourth question asks, and is answered, in the same way but deals with the *last* outcome. Respondents are then asked for the number of times they have experienced each outcome in the last twelve months. They are also asked if they have ever been pregnant on purpose, and if so, when this happened for the last time. The remaining four questions are the same as those asked of the males, dealing with contraception, pregnancy "wantedness," and future plans. With this series of pregnancy history questions, the completed response rate is higher than with any other series we have explored, and internal consistency is good.

What problems are there with other formats? Essentially, it should be noted that we did not begin this series by asking the respondents an over-arching question, "Have you ever been pregnant?" Based on previous studies, there is the danger that one such question might incorrectly skip respondents over the rest of the pregnancy section when, indeed, there was reason for them to complete it. This is because, to many young women, pregnancy is the equivalent of "having a baby" and the other possible outcomes do not come to mind. Asking whether the respondent has experienced each outcome separately and serially, in the beginning of the pregnancy series, minimizes linguistic confusion.

Therefore, this format maximizes the chances of a complete response. Incomplete responses confound the entire series, and lead to the loss of valuable information. Additional problems in understanding pregnancy data will be discussed in chapter 5.

The series of questions on pregnancy history are much simpler for younger students. There are three components: ever pregnant (or ever impregnated), number of times this has occurred in the last twelve months, and outcome the last time. Since fertility histories are much briefer for youngsters still in the seventh and eighth grades, the possibility of losing valuable information is small, and information on events before the age of eleven or twelve will probably be unreliable even if the questions are included. Clearly, the need for brevity is a pressing one for younger readers; if a long series of compli-cated questions can be omitted without a serious loss of data, that is much to be desired.

Some additional behavioral questions are asked, not for evaluation but for background purposes or basic research. For example, there are questions on the sexual behavior of friends of the respondent, and older students are asked about pregnancy among their friends, as well. All students are asked if they are presently "going with" a boy/girl and if so, for how long; they are asked his or her age. Different dating patterns among teens may be relevant not only to their other sexual conduct, but in turn to behaviors that are similarly age related. One might ask, for example, does a young girl who is dating a considerably older partner run the danger of being involved in levels of substance use generally associated with later teenage years?

An attempt is made to explore whether the students have ever had a venereal disease, and if so, what type. Older students are asked when this occurred for the last time. The data look unreliable. Comparing this infor-mation to what is known about rates of sexually transmitted diseases in the same population (data often available from other local clinics or the health department), the reported rates are much too low. It appears that this is an area about which few, if any, conclusions can be drawn from self-reported questionnaire data, except, perhaps, the fact that young people are sadly unaware of their own sexual health status. This negative finding has programmatic implications for education and medical service, but does not suggest that the area can profitably be explored in survey instruments if time is of the essence.

One-half of the older sample and all the younger students are asked some questions about substance use. This includes whether they smoke cigarettes (they respond by checking how many a day), when they began to smoke, and how old they were at the time (the younger students are not asked the last portion of the question). They are also asked whether they drink beer or wine, drink hard liquor, smoke pot, or use any other street drugs; in each case, they are asked how many times they used that substance during the previous month. This series on substance use has been interesting, but is clearly minimal. It will have to be expanded for programs with strong components in this area. Many models exist for intensive exploration of substance use, either as a combined set of variables or focusing separately on alcohol, drugs, or tobacco. These can be obtained through the Alcohol, Drug Abuse and Mental Health Administration of the National Institutes of Health, and therefore will not be discussed further here.

The other half of the split sample of older students, and all the younger students, are asked if they have ever discussed a series of topics with their parents or friends. These include menstruation, pregnancy risk, being a teen parent, birth control, and venereal disease. This is the same half of the split sample whose questions on sex education and household structure were described on page 49. They are also asked what time they have to be home at night, on weekdays and on weekends, as an indicator of parental guidance or control. Thus some insight may be obtained into the relationship between the source of sexual information, household structure, parental behavior in relation to their teenagers, and the behaviors and attitudes reflected in the rest of the questionnaire.

All younger students are asked some information about their activities outside of school: sports, books, television, church groups. All ninth- through twelfth-grade students are asked whether they plan to marry someone they are presently dating. There are many areas of these sorts one would wish to explore, but once again, the voracious appetites of researchers need to be kept within the bounds of strict time limitations. Questions have to be restricted to behaviors the researchers and the service providers, together, feel are most likely to impinge on the students' need for the program, and on its potential or actual utilization.

Program Use

In all rounds after the first, the baseline round, questionnaires for the schools in which the program is being evaluated require a series of questions to ascertain who used which of the program's services. These questionnaires should reflect the shape of the particular service model, so that the various components of its design are tapped and, if possible, individually assessed. In the Hopkins program, for example, that includes exploring utilization in both program sites, the school and the clinic, and it includes educational and medical, individual and group services. Questions on utilization might change over the life of the program, with the researchers adding and subtracting variables as the program unfolds. There is less reason to keep these questions similar, a rigid demand which puts stringent limits on one's ability to modify the instrument in the areas we discussed previously. Unless one is specifically trying to assess usage of a particular component over time, some variation in the questions is acceptable and only the final evaluation instrument needs to be truly exhaustive.

Questions relative to the school component include, initially, the basic fact of program recognition. In the Hopkins program, this included: do the students know that there are providers from the program to whom they can talk privately in the school? Have the providers ever talked to their classes? Have they, personally, ever talked in school with these providers, and for what reasons have they done so? Other questions, even from earlier rounds, deal with the use or non-use of the program clinic. Thus, in all questionnaires, students are asked if they have ever gone to the program clinic, and if so, why they went there and how many times they have attended. This was asked as an open-ended question in some surveys, but since answers are generally grouped for analysis, they are grouped here in the final instrument (never, one to two, and three or more). In earlier rounds, when the questions are more exploratory, and are aimed at program improvement rather than at summative evaluation, there may be a place for additional open-ended questions on the reason for clinic attendance, by whom they were accompanied, and what they "liked best." The last question, in our case, was expanded considerably as the program progressed, with longer checklists identifying the likes and dislikes of the students. Similarly, those who have never been to the clinic, or who had but were no longer attending, were asked on a checklist to indicate why. Respondents who attended other family planning clinics or physicians since the program clinic was available to them were given a checklist as well. In the last two years of the program, respondents were asked where they last received the method of birth control they were presently using and what method it was. They were asked how important they believed it was that program providers speak in their classrooms and be available in school to help students get to the program clinic. They were asked how much the program had changed their feelings about getting pregnant (or impregnating a girl) while in school, and about the use of birth control. The questions retained in the final instrument and presented in appendix C, show the breadth of variables that can add to our understanding of program involvement.

The final questionnaire, however, adds an important dimension. An attempt is made to understand the degree to which the program facility *substituted* for other sites, and the degree to which it actually changed contraceptive behavior. Thus, questions are asked on the timing of first attendance at the program facility, and males and females alike are asked about contraception obtained in the year before, and since, attendance at the program clinic. Of course, it is possible that the students do not have a source of contraception, either because they use a method that does not require medical advice, because they do not use contraception at all, and/or because they do not engage in coitus. For those who do, however, an attempt is made to understand the reasons for their choice of their regular source of contraception, whatever it is, and if that source is not the program facility, what special reasons there may be for that decision.

These questions, perhaps more than any others in the questionnaire, will reflect the type of program being evaluated. As already suggested, consistency between questionnaires may not be as important as an emerging set of variables that help the providers and the researchers to understand the interaction between the students and the program—its offerings and its staff. If the program administrators are seriously interested in utilizing the results of the earlier questionnaires in updating their design, they should have a large role in developing this section of the survey instrument. A measure of the sensitivity of the staff to the students they serve will be the feedback mechanisms they develop for utilizing these results in constructive ways to improve their services.

Since no such offerings are made to students in the schools used as controls, none of these questions are asked. There may, however, be some counseling components in the school's regular program, or some health initiatives that are a part of routine school health services. It is generally of interest to school administrators to know the extent to which their students are utilizing these services, and it is also useful to the researchers to understand the level of parallel activity in a school which is not involved in the special project. In the non-program schools' baseline questionnaire, therefore, students were asked whether they had talked, personally, with a school counselor about contraception, pregnancy, and/or parenting. A more complete series of questions on this topic should be designed whenever the control schools offer guidance programs or health services, however limited they may be compared to the experimental program.

Special Topics

We have indicated how important it is to prune the questionnaire wherever possible, in the interests of readability and simplicity, as well as time. However, as previously indicated, there is a large section on program use which is omitted or minimized in the survey instrument used for the non-program schools. This may allow time for the exploration of some special topic(s). Furthermore, even in the program schools, senior high school students may have time to complete some extra questions; they can be added *if* the variables will not be seriously affected by the selection process: slower readers may not have time to complete them. These extra topics may be included as an integral part of the questionnaire, but placed at the end, or may be in the nature of a small, auxiliary questionnaire which is attached to the basic instrument for those who have time to complete it, or handed out to respondents as they finish working on the basic survey instrument. To maximize its value, however, it should be kept *with* the basic survey, so it can be analyzed in the context of the same student's overall response.

An example of the first type of addendum is a series of questions added to the final survey, for all females who have had a baby, to assess the relationship between schooling, child care, and the role of the baby's father. These questions, which appear in appendix C, are not sufficient to explore the relationship between school dropout and child care in any detail, but rather provide background information for future designs that can investigate the subject in depth. Other researchers will wish to pose similar areas for future exploration, and can usefully utilize any time which even a few respondents may have to begin to understand how best to research new areas. The insights may turn out to be useful in the evaluation, but even if they are not, they can advance the field by preparing the way for future investigations.

The second type of exploration was a separate, one-page questionnaire given to students in earlier rounds if and when they completed the original instrument. It explored utilization of the media, and dealt with students' perceptions of what TV shows seem to be saying about sex, pregnancy risk, and contraception. It asks for numbers of hours a week spent watching TV, listening to the radio or to records and tapes, for the frequency with which they watch specific types of TV shows, and for information on what, if any, parental restrictions apply to the TV shows they are permitted to watch. Students are asked their favorite TV programs, radio stations, music, and magazines; an attempt can be made to relate this information to the sexual, contraceptive, and pregnancy behavior reported by the same respondents. Although, once again, the appetites of the researchers should be controlled, this opportunity is an important one, because these types of ancillary questionnaires do not need to be repeated at every survey administration. Since the results are suggestive only, researchers can deal with different topics at different times, and can add considerably to the richness of the research.

AIDS: New Variables to Explore

Since this program was conceived in 1981, a new area of serious concern has made it advisable to open new areas of investigation in surveys such as these. We need to know the likelihood of the spread of acquired immuno-deficiency syndrome, or, more specifically, of HIV infection, in our adolescent populations. The seriousness of the epidemic may influence potential opponents to permit researchers to ask questions that they previously found unacceptable. On the other hand, adding questions on homosexual behaviors may increase opposition by small, hostile minorities. Once again, school boards, principals, parents, teachers, and communities will need time and information to help them to understand the compelling need for such data from young people at high risk. In addition to the questions on drug abuse which we included, specific information on needle-administered drugs should be obtained. In the area of homosexual behavior, two different concepts need to be addressed. One explores the young person's concept of himself— Does he see himself as gay? The second has to do with the occurrence, at any time, of sexual contact with a member of his own sex. Same-sex contact is a great deal more common than the self-concept "homosexuality." The former says nothing about current behavior and, in fact, little of behavior at any time. Using the self-concept as the behavior would yield an underestimate of the actual risk, because early experimentation would not be tapped. To round out the picture of risk status, it might be advisable to include a question on the occurrence of a blood transfusion between 1979 and 1985, although it is very unlikely that the self-report of adolescents would yield an accurate estimate. There are probably better sources for this information than aggregate survey data.

Data Preparation

Questionnaires were distributed to the classroom teachers in packets. The teachers were responsible for returning every questionnaire they received, those that were completed and those that were blank (see chapter 1). Questionnaires were kept in their packets, by classroom, in order to assign identification numbers by classroom. These were six-digit numbers. The first three digits were printed in advance on the questionnaires; they represent the school, the round, and the questionnaire type (age group and gender) but do not identify individuals at all. The last three digits, filled in later in consecutive order for each school/round/questionnaire type, make it possible to identify a particular questionnaire during the cleaning and analysis phase. By maintaining a list of the identification numbers assigned to questionnaires from each classroom, the researchers are permitted to identify respondents from different educational levels within the grade (if such exist), which may for some evaluations be of considerable importance.

The next major step is coding the questionnaires; this process will always have to take place unless the instrument has been designed to be electronically scanned, a rather complex and often expensive task. It would be well worth the investment of time and effort if the same instrument, with very minimal change, were to be used for large numbers of students. Hand-coding can be carried out in several ways: the information can be transferred from the questionnaires to codesheets, or can be coded on the questionnaires themselves; although many questionnaires are precoded, so that data entry can be accomplished directly from the questionnaire, that is extremely difficult to do with interlocking, complex questions such as those contained in the sample. In any case, a codebook must be written for each questionnaire type, describing skip patterns, and making it possible to identify inappropriate, inconsistent, and incomplete information. During the coding process, skilled coders and editors need to search for inconsistencies and, where possible, correct questionnaires when it is absolutely clear from the context that a simple omission has been made. (Some researchers prefer to do this during the data cleaning process.) This should be done with extreme caution, as it is better to record no answer at all than to attribute an incorrect response. Ideally, the questionnaires and coding forms should be reedited by a second person, who can check the coding and concentrate on the whole questionnaire. This makes it possible to recognize major problems which may emerge. A process should also be designed in advance for resolving discrepancies between the first and second editors. For example, one supervising researcher can be responsible for final coding decisions. This long and arduous coding process has many advantages, not the least of which is that an initial cleaning of the data by at least two people has occurred before the information is computerized. The questionnaires can be evaluated in advance, and assigned a questionnaire "quality value," which in our case ranged from 1 (best) to 3 (poor); fortunately, very few questionnaires fell into the last category. The major disadvantage of the process described here is that it is extremely slow, time consuming, and therefore expensive.

The same check/double-check method should be used in the keypunching process. The current study, employing separate codesheets, delivered only the sheets to the keypuncher, maintaining the questionnaires in locked files. All the keypunched material was 100 percent verified by a second keypuncher.

Whatever techniques are used for coding and keypunching these elaborate questionnaires, a thorough cleaning of the computerized raw data records must precede analysis. An efficient computer program for frequencies and tables can cut the costs of this operation, but, unfortunately, cannot cut the time that must be invested. (A program called *Select*, written by John

Karat at The Johns Hopkins University School of Hygiene and Public Health, was invaluable in this process.) The various steps recommended for data cleaning are listed in appendix D. Essentially there are three steps, which involve looking at (1) frequencies, (2) crosstabulations, and (3) comparison of ages and dates. In the current study, in addition to all of these computer checks, each step of which led to a return to the original documents, an even more thorough check was made of the pregnancy variables. Because these involved an important outcome measure, and because they involved inter- locking dates, outcomes, and often histories, they were too important and complex to leave to the regular cleaning process. Finally, a systems file must be created, so that all rounds can be matched in format, and analysis can compare similar measures across the survey rounds without undue complication.

Clearly, the coding and cleaning process must be done meticulously, by data handlers who are precise, accurate, and consistent. Any ambiguity that remains in any of the responses may be difficult to pinpoint once the systems file is created; at that point what is on the computer replaces what is on the questionnaire. The value of the final analysis is as dependent on the decisions made during the coding and cleaning phase as it is on the initial design of the questionnaire.

Notes toward a Simplified Survey Instrument

The variables presented in this long discussion clearly go far beyond the barest needs for program evaluation. They add to the richness of our un- derstanding of the patient population, hence to our ability to define their needs, but they add up to an instrument that may go well beyond the staffing and financial capacities of many programs, even programs that desire effec- tive evaluation. What is the minimum requirement for such an effort?

Whatever the area of health service, a certain amount of demographic/ background information is required. This certainly includes age, grade, race, and, for reasons we have detailed above, the grade at which the student entered the school, and the school from which the student came. Information on household structure may or may not be needed; similarly, information on the behavior of siblings or other peers may appear relevant. Secondly, some minimal information on knowledge ought to be included. This section will be larger in proportion to the importance of an educational component in the project, but even in a strictly health service program, it is useful to know the degree to which misinformation influences student participation or compliance. As we have indicated, attitudinal data are somewhat less reliable and are often at odds with behavior; as interesting an area as this is to explore, in a minimal document it may have to be eliminated. It may be that all that can remain of an attitudinal nature are the students' perceptions of services in the field encompassed by the experimental project. This information, although not essential for a summative, or outcome, evaluation, is crucial to an understanding of the process by which the intervention worked.

In evaluating a program that seeks to change behavior, the most important area in the questionnaire, and that which must not be shortchanged, is the section covering the behaviors which the program seeks to affect. These need to be carefully described, asking input from professional providers with long experience in the field. Using the correct idiom is essential here, as it is throughout the survey. It is of particular importance to cover all aspects of the respondents' histories in the area under investigation. Thus, and only thus, will the material be at hand for the analyses discussed in the next chapter, and the complex task of assessing change in personal behaviors be accomplished.

5
Problems in Evaluation Analysis

With data in hand, collected *before* the program is in place and again at some *follow-up* period or periods, the raw materials for the evaluation are in place. The structure has not yet been built; methods employed during the analysis phase can still determine how strong the assessment will be—how accurate and how sensitive, and how credible its findings.

Exposure Groups, Grades, and Age

One of the issues that plague evaluation in a school setting is handling the question of age at a time of life when age is so sensitive a variable. Adolescence, perhaps more than any phase of life with the exception of infancy, is characterized by change. Even in the absence of special programs, growth, development, learning, and behavioral transitions are to be expected. It is essential, therefore, to know the age distributions of groups we seek to compare; if one group is significantly older than another we expect more sexual activity, more substance use, more knowledge, all differences that are highly age dependent. Normal changes with age should not be confused with the effects of interventions, as difficult as it may be to keep them apart. When we look at behaviors *within* grade, it is easier to separate program effects. Although ages and grades may not match perfectly for all students, grades are nonetheless good surrogates for age, and since we need to control by grade for reasons of exposure, it becomes useful to do so in order to separate age and program effects, as well.

Furthermore, controlling by grade allows one, at a glance, to understand the differences in program effects by age—a particularly important area of study when planning where, or at what age level, programs can most effectively be conducted. Figure 5–1 shows graphically how much information is conveyed when the survey results are tabulated by grade. It illustrates one variable, attendance at a contraceptive clinic, by grade, among boys and

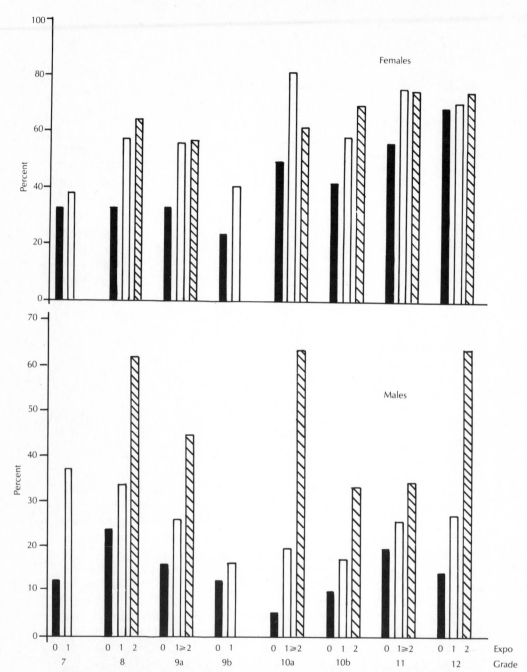

Figure 5–1. Percent of Sexually Active Junior and Senior High School Black Males and Females Ever Having Been to a Birth Control Clinic, by Years of Exposure to a Pregnancy Prevention Program and by Grade

girls at the program schools. Note that the improvement is much greater for younger than older students, and greater for males than for females. Many substantive findings are conveyed when the results of the study are displayed in this way. There is one obvious problem. It is hard to sum up program effects when reporting them in so many individual subgroups: we are given eight separate comparisons when, ideally, there would be one single summary statistic that could intuitively be understood.

In chapter 3 we discussed the relationship between grades, rounds, and exposures, and suggested that the appropriate comparisons for the evaluation were between exposure groups rather than rounds. Figure 5–2, adapted from figure 3–1, in chapter 3, illustrates the fact that, when distributing the findings by grade, several grade/exposure cells are not available for comparison. We note, for example, how in a junior high school, seventh graders can only have one year's exposure to a program no matter how long it is in place. The absence of certain cells—in this example, the absence of two- or three-year exposures for seventh graders—makes comparisons most accurate when comparing within grade. In each comparison, then, one can use only exposures relevant to the particular grade level. Thus there are not only substantive but methodological indications for controlling by grade.

Figure 5–2 shows graphically how many cells would be missing were we to sum, horizontally, across grades. Obviously, simple totals would be misleading; groups with *longer exposure* tend to be older than those with

	Junior High School			Senior High School					Total	Adjusted Total
Exposure	7	8	9a	9b	10a	10b	11	12		
0										
1										X
2	X			X					X	
3	X			X		X			X	
	OR									
≥2	X			X					X	

Figure 5–2. Relation between Exposures, Grades, and Totals

shorter exposure, since within each school, they include only the older grades. (In the case of the control schools, no such problem exists, because all grades are treated as "zero exposure" groups; baseline and follow-up comparisons both utilize all grade/school groups.)

What would be the effect of the age discrepancies in the experimental schools if one summed across grades and made a simple comparison of everybody available before and everybody available after some specific period, exposure zero and exposure two, for example? The most obvious effects would be that more students would smoke, more would have had sex, more would have knowledge of certain relevant information after than before, and it would be difficult to know what portion of that change was attributable to the program, if any. After all, the exposure two group will be older, and more older students have had sex or smoked than younger students, and knowledge tends to increase, not decrease, over time. These are, generally speaking, cumulative rates. Therefore, comparisons within grade are much more easily interpreted and much more accurate than summary measures. Nonetheless, when considering or reporting on the findings, simpler summary measures are generally required. Eight separate comparisons for our eight school/grade groups, for example, would be seen as cumbersome and even obfuscating. How can a summary measure be generated that accounts for differentials in age distribution and expresses all the information available on true program effects?

In our case, the problem was addressed by standardizing the follow-up periods in the program schools on the grade distribution of the students who answered the question in the baseline survey. When grades are missing, an "adjusted total" is computed *omitting* those grades from the baseline data as well, so that the comparisons will be made between total samples with similar age distributions. (Standardizing is a simple process described in many statistics textbooks.)

Using this procedure, exposures of one year are standardized to control for the numbers in each grade, but *not* adjusted by the omission of any grades at all. This is because all grades, in spring, have been exposed for one year to a program in place for that time. However, for exposures of two or more years, some grade or grades will need to be omitted from the baseline data in order to make the samples match; the grades that are omitted in the adjusted totals are those that are missing from the follow-up data because no students in that grade could have been exposed for the relevant length of time.

In addition to controlling for exposures, this method allows one to correct for differences in the percents of students attending each grade when the several rounds of the survey are administered. Since all exposures are standardized on the distribution of the baseline data in the program schools, accurate comparisons can be made. In the *control schools,* both the baseline and follow-up periods are also standardized on the baseline distribution in the *program schools,* in order to avoid any possible difference in grade distributions at either the earlier or later time period between the experimental and control sites.

Finally, the adjusted total allows one to correct for any local problems that may arise in a specific setting, on a specific day of survey administration. Thus, should one grade be out on a trip, should seniors already be absent in large numbers in anticipation of graduation, in other words should any grade in the sample be contaminated in any way, that grade can be omitted without invalidating the study, as long as the grade that is omitted from the follow-up survey is omitted from the baseline data as well.

It may have occurred to the reader of the preceding paragraphs that there is, indeed, an age differential between those surveyed in the baseline and follow-up rounds if the baseline is collected in fall and the follow-ups are administered in spring. We indicated that spring follow-ups are useful because they allow us to capture students who will be leaving the schools. Unfortunately, given the nature of school systems, it is unlikely that there will be a chance to collect baseline data the spring *before* the program begins. Schools will rarely know long enough in advance that a program is planned for fall to allow the researchers to be prepared for data collection before the end of the previous school year. Therefore, in most cases, the student sample will be slightly older at the time of the follow-up surveys than it was at the time the baseline information was collected.

Generally, the age differential in this case will have little effect on variables that are not highly age dependent because it will be a difference of only six, seven, or eight months. It could, however, have some effect on those variables that reflect cumulative experience, variables such as percent ever sexually active, percent ever using specific substances, and so on. As will be described in the following, we suggest the use of life table analysis wherever appropriate to correct for the age difference in variables such as these. This technique permits us to measure the percentages of students to adopt certain behaviors by specific, exact ages, rather than using grade as a surrogate for age as we do when characteristics are less sensitive to exact age. We do not have to guess which characteristics these are; having so much information, calculated by grade, allows us to see immediately which variables are particularly dependent on age, by comparing the graded information in the baseline data.

Examining differences by grade before and after exposure has the additional benefit of helping to elucidate changes the program has made in the relationship between a characteristic and age: for example, does the program make younger girls come to a clinic more promptly after first sex, and thus reduce the difference between younger and older females, and does it therefore reduce the additional risks of conception usually experienced by younger, sexually active girls? Similarly, the technique answers questions in other fields of inquiry: do younger boys respond less well, or better, than older boys to drug prevention programs? In which group is the program better able to lower the level of alcohol use? Do comprehensive health clinics reach one age group better than another? Is there an age group they do not appear to be reaching?

It should be clear from the preceding paragraphs that using controls by grade adds a great deal to the richness of the study whether the evaluation is used to upgrade the program's design or to evaluate its final impact. When a summary statistic is required, the procedure described here makes it methodologically sound to sum across appropriate grades, both to control for differences in program exposure and to account for changes which may occur in the relative sizes of different grades in any of the schools in the course of the program.

Simple Cross-Sectional Analysis

The raw data from each survey, in essence, give us a snapshot of the school populations at a single point of time. What can one do with these raw data to develop an accurate picture, to examine the results? The simplest measures are percents, which allow us to determine how many respondents out of the total agreed with the proposed attitude, knew a particular fact, or experienced a specific behavior. Percentages are easily understood, and useful for exploring the distribution of a characteristic in a population, and for comparing that distribution between groups. They are easy to calculate (programs to obtain them are found in most computer statistical packages). Univariate and bivariate distributions are important and will take the researcher a long way in carrying out the evaluation.

When researchers have asked many related questions, it is sometimes desirable to examine the results in the form of one summary number, rather than attempting to interpret each finding separately. It is easier to digest one statement about one characteristic than many. To do this, an *index* can be created. There are many ways to combine results; books have been written that discuss only these techniques. In the simplest kind of index, responses that represent a single dimension are combined into a score or grade. Thus, in the Hopkins project, a knowledge index was created from ten questions about contraception, pregnancy risk, and abortion. Each correct answer was given a score of one; all other answers, including no answer, were given a score of zero, and the ten scores were added. The value of the knowledge index ranged from zero to ten, with a score of ten indicating that the respondent answered all the questions correctly.

A second type of index is a slightly more eclectic form of the first, combining characteristics that may not be as formally related but have an intuitive relationship one with the other. Again in the Hopkins study, attitudes supportive of adolescent parenting were looked at in such a way. Whether they were drawn from true/false questions, multiple choice questions, or agree/disagree questions, any variable that tapped the respondent's belief that childbearing during the teen years was or was not a "good thing" was included in this summary variable, which gave a score of one to respondents holding any attitude supportive of adolescent childbearing, and a zero to those holding none. If, in utilizing these characteristics, one is making the assumption that there is an association between these variables, the careful researcher may wish to employ some method of cluster analysis, to be certain the variables are really related.

A more complicated example of indexing might be the development of a summary indicator such as we created to measure the level of substance abuse in the last twelve months. This was formed by weighting the frequency of use of a substance by an estimate of the degree to which that substance is considered dangerous, and then summing over all available substances. Clearly, in order to do this, some outside information is required, because, although the frequency of use is drawn directly from the survey data, the assignment of weights to each substance depends on expert input from the field.

Another type of measure that is frequently useful in examining survey results is the *cumulative percentage* of respondents who experience a behavior over a given period of time. This observation can be treated as a snapshot too, because once the number is developed it can function as a picture of a characteristic at the present point in time. However, the cumulative percentage is most accurately calculated using life table methodology, which allows one to observe the history of the behavior over time. This is a much more complex task, as will be discussed in the following sections.

Analyzing Behavioral Histories

In chapter 4, we stress the importance of historical information when trying to understand the onset of key behaviors, and the patterns of these behaviors over time. Thus, in a drug program, for example, it might be necessary to establish an age of first use of a range of substances, a level of use for some specified period or periods, increases or decreases or even cessations in use, and so on. The construction of the survey instrument that must capture these developments has been addressed before. Here we are interested more directly in problems in the interpretation of the response, and the analytic methods that help us handle this historical information. A particularly challenging variable will be used to illustrate the complexity of the task.

Measuring Pregnancy Rates

Although it may appear that a conception is a reasonably straightforward event, measuring the frequency of its occurrence is a complicated and difficult process. We focus here on the methodology for females, since this variable must ultimately be used as a direct measure of a pregnancy prevention program's impact. (Measuring the occurrence of impregnation by males is even more of a challenge. The data collected from males are generally of lower quality, and there are no data available for external checks.)

First, one has to determine the objective of the program. Is it to prevent pregnancy? Is it to prevent a particular pregnancy outcome such as childbearing? Or is it to do both? Next, one has to decide how to ask the questions that best measure that goal. For example, will it give better data to ask about individual pregnancy outcomes, or is the overall question, "Have you ever been pregnant?" preferable? As discussed in chapter 4, we feel that data are of a higher quality when respondents are asked about individual pregnancy outcomes. In doing this, however, some compromises may have to be made; unless all possible outcomes are included, using individual outcomes may cause one to miss some pregnancies. For example, in the interest of economy we omit stillbirths, since they occur so infrequently. A rare pregnancy may well be missed.

Another consideration is how to establish the date of the respondent's pregnancy. Does one ask the date of the outcome, the date of conception, the length of gestation? We believe that the most reliable information comes from asking the date of the outcome, an event for which the respondent's recall is probably accurate. It is then possible to estimate the date of conception by making assumptions about gestation (for example, nine months for a live birth and three months for an abortion or miscarriage). The researcher may wish to ask the length of gestation and the conception date and decide afterwards whether the information is valid. However, in the interest of limiting the number of questions on the questionnaire, we do not recommend doing so. We ask only the date of the outcome, believing the respondent much more likely to recall that date than either conception or gestation. Overall, the margin of error will not be large if only that single piece of information is obtained, no larger than the possible error if the respondent is asked to recall two dates and the researcher is forced to reconcile discrepancies in that recall. This issue is particularly important if a researcher is interested in the number of pregnancies in a certain time period. For example, the number of *outcomes* in the last twelve months could be different from the number of *conceptions* in the last twelve months. A female could have conceived fourteen months before the survey, hence before the period of interest, but still have had the pregnancy outcome in the relevant period.

Pregnancy is the most difficult parameter to assess for several reasons. First, like other behaviors, "ever pregnant" proportions are cumulative. Thus, the number experiencing the behavior cannot decrease if the same females are asked about this behavior at two points in time. Second, the reporting of outcomes other than live birth may be problematic. *Miscarriages* are not well reported, particularly by young females, because early miscarriages may be missed; in fact, with irregular cycles, inexperience, and no expectation of pregnancy, miscarriages at any gestation may not be identified as such. However, after awareness of pregnancy and its symptoms is heightened by an educational program, young women may recall experiencing them, and the rate of their occurrence may artifactually appear to increase. As for *abortions*, young women may not call induced abortions "pregnancies," or may not admit that they occurred. They may be more willing to admit to abortions after the program, with the same artifactual result. Similarly, the statement that one is *"pregnant now"* may be ambiguous; it may be a guess if a pregnancy test has not been performed. It is hard to know if one is counting diagnosed pregnancies or "pregnancy scares." We know that the latter number is much higher than the former. Third, pregnancy and school attendance may be related. This contributes to an underestimate of pregnancy rates from aggregate school data, especially if a high proportion of recently pregnant girls are absent on the day of the survey or if females who get pregnant have dropped out of school. However, as shown in chapter 3, if these proportions do not change over time, it can be assumed that they will not affect the comparison of rates over time.

Finally, pregnancy takes longer than other behaviors to be affected by a program. If one wants to calculate a twelve-month birth rate to determine whether or not births have been affected by the program, an additional nine program months must be added in order to prevent conception first—one year plus nine months back from birth to conception, for a total of twenty-one program months. By the same logic, it would take a minimum of fifteen months to affect an abortion rate (twelve months plus three months). Therefore, it is unrealistic to expect to see a measurable difference in pregnancy rates after a program has been in place only one year. These relationships must be understood or the early findings in a pregnancy prevention program could actually be misleading; for example, if births are being replaced with abortions, both pregnancies and abortions might actually appear to increase initially due to the shorter gestation of abortions. Or, when both childbearing *and* abortion are declining, abortions would appear to come down first because there may not yet have been time to observe the decline in births.

The simplest pregnancy rate to calculate is the number of pregnant girls divided by the number of girls (or sexually active girls), with both the numerator and the denominator referring to the same group and the same time period. For greatest accuracy, the number of *conceptions* should be used in that estimate, as indicated previously. Alternatively, the numerator can be limited to a particular pregnancy outcome—for example, a live birth.

There are two possible figures to use for the denominator of such a pregnancy rate. One is the number of *all* females in the study and the other is the number of females actually at risk of pregnancy—that is, those who are sexually active. If *all females* are in the denominator, changes in rates may be due to changes in the proportions of girls who are sexually active, rather than in the proportions of sexually active girls getting pregnant. It may be seen as an advantage, however, that pregnancies are then related to the entire population, and that a change in the pregnancy rate reflects both the behaviors that impact upon that rate. On the other hand, using the number of *sexually active females* as the denominator is advantageous because it limits the proportion to only those eligible to contribute to the numerator, and changes can be attributed directly to the behavior of sexually active young women—for example, their use of contraception or frequency of intercourse. (Of course, to limit the denominator to the sexually active, one is required to collect the appropriate information, but that is probably of interest in any case.)

Simple rates like these are useful in that they are easy to collect data for, to calculate, and to understand. However, they tell nothing about the risk of the event over time. The statistical method of life table analysis can be employed to examine that risk. Life tables allow for the maximum amount of information to be used on each respondent while controlling for the interval of observation. A discussion of this methodology follows.

Life Tables

Life tables are an important statistical technique in the Hopkins evaluation model. Why are they used? They are used to examine the probability of an event *over time* or by an *exact age*. They allow us to employ in the analysis the maximum amount of information collected on each individual, because when using this method everyone need not be observed for exactly the same amount of time. This section will not attempt to "teach" life table methodology. It will seek only to explain the technique so the purpose of life tables in evaluation research can be understood. We hope it will serve as a basis for an understanding of life table programs in standard statistical packages, and will help ensure the collection of the necessary variables.

In the life table technique, all respondents in the denominator are "entered" at the initial time (or age) chosen to start the table. Two pieces of information are then needed for each respondent in order to calculate a life table: (1) why the respondent is "exiting" the table; is she removed at the occurrence of the event of interest (known as the "terminal event"—for example, a clinic visit, a first drink, a conception), or is she withdrawn because the end of the study's observation period has been reached? (2) The length of observation, usually from the beginning of the table (an age or a time) to the occurrence of the exit event.

In the evaluation of the Hopkins program, life tables were used to examine, for example, the probability of first having sexual intercourse by a given age, and the probability of attending a clinic or becoming pregnant by a certain time after first exposure. In other programs they could elucidate the ages of onset of certain substance, delinquent, or school behaviors, or the time between use of a substance and attendance at a prevention program. We will illustrate the use of life tables by describing how we calculated the probability of sexual onset among females.

All females in the survey entered the table at one age, before any of them were sexually active. They stayed in the table until they reached the age at which they experienced this "terminal event," their first sexual intercourse, or until the age at which they took the survey (that is, they were withdrawn from the table when no more data were available, at a time when they were still virgins). One could then calculate the cumulative percentage of females who had had sexual intercourse by the time they reached each exact age.

With life table methodology, one has to select carefully who to include in the comparison. In this case, we could include only those who had *not had sexual intercourse before their exposure to the program,* among those females who were exposed to the program. It would not make sense to measure the effect of the program on sexual onset among those who had already experienced intercourse. Second, we had to choose the duration of *exposure* to the program in which we were interested; we chose to examine the probability of sexual onset among those with one, two, or three years of exposure. Third, we had to consider the *age distribution* of females exposed to the program for these lengths of time. In other words, most of those exposed to the program for three years had to be at least fifteen at the time of Round IV, because the program only started with girls of approximately age twelve. Thus the three-year exposure life table was limited to those fifteen and older, whereas the one-year exposure life table had no age restriction. Fourth, a *comparable group* had to be selected from the baseline data. We used females who were the same age for the same durations of exposure. Of course, in the baseline data (or in the control schools) no one was "exposed" to the program. Nonetheless, to compare their ages of sexual onset they had to be followed for identical periods of time. How long was that? It was the number of years before the baseline survey *equal to* the number of years of program exposure for the group to which they were being compared. The data from the control schools were treated in the same way as the data from the program schools' baseline surveys. In all cases only females who had not had sexual intercourse before the beginning of the period were included.

Pregnancy life tables are more complex than those previously described because in the course of time, more young women initiate coitus and have to be added to the group being studied. We use a life table methodology known as "increment-decrement," in a procedure which we will describe briefly so that it can be replicated by the experienced programmer. As females became sexually active and/or pregnant after their exposure to the program they have to be added to and taken from the table. Females are entered into the table at the time of their first sexual intercourse. If they have had sexual intercourse before being exposed to the program, they are entered at the beginning of the table (unless they are pregnant at that time). If sexual onset occurred after first program exposure, they are added to the table in the month in which they began sex. They are terminated from the table when a conception occurred, or withdrawn at the time of the survey. Conception dates for pregnancy outcomes are estimated from the dates of the outcome, assuming a nine-month gestation for a live birth, and a three-month gestation for abortions and miscarriages. Conception dates for the currently pregnant are calculated using the current gestation.

We used several different lengths of exposure, which were derived from the dates of the surveys and the opening of the program clinic. Others will wish to select exposures which relate to the particulars of their own programs. Once selected, the same lengths of time must be used for the program baseline survey and for the control schools. (For the pregnancy analysis, we used Round II data as baseline for the program school since the Round II, III, and IV surveys were all done at the same time of year. This made for greater accuracy in these delicate calculations because it ensured comparable age distributions between the baseline and the exposure groups. In these and all other adjustments, we made a point of erring in the direction that tended to minimize rather than maximize positive program effects.)

One problem with estimating pregnancy rates, as discussed in the preceding, is the possibility of missing information in the aggregate data on pregnant girls who leave school after being exposed to the program. Although it is universally difficult to retrieve any information on those who drop out of the school system, it may be possible to collect information, as we were able to do in Baltimore, on a large and important subset: those who attend a special school for pregnant girls. In our case, the school was willing and able to provide us with lists of entrants who had come from the program and control schools, including their dates of confinement, the dates on which they entered and left the special school, and the school to which they returned. Based on this information, used in conjunction with school lists (see chapter 6), we could determine whether they were exposed to the program before they became pregnant and were enrolled in the school for pregnant girls at the time of the survey. If so, they were added to the appropriate life tables. Their lengths of program exposure were calculated from the information we were given. Their dates of conception were estimated using dates of confinement, assuming a nine-month gestation. It is possible to utilize information of this kind even if these young women are not available to answer the questionnaire, and thus cannot supply all the information available on the other respondents. In this case, their dates of first intercourse were estimated, using the assumption that these students had initiated sexual intercourse thirteen months before they became pregnant; this period was selected because thirteen months was the average delay between first coitus and conception observed among all the pregnant students for whom we had complete documentation in both the program and non-program schools. (The same assumption was made for pregnant girls in the aggregate data for whom a date of first intercourse was missing.) Thus, the most important single group of "transfers"—the group with a pregnancy rate of 100 percent—was included in our estimates. Locating and finding a way to do this is a challenge to evaluators of other types of programs, as well; the assumptions one has to make in order to incorporate them are very minor compared to the possible error that could be caused by leaving them out, if they comprise a significant proportion of the relevant cases.

Using Self-Reported "Utilization" Information

We devoted a good deal of attention in chapter 3 to the process of establishing the size of the student population in a study school. This number, as we indicated, is the denominator used to calculate the proportion of all students receiving any given service. The numerator, or the actual count of services, is usually drawn from the actual records of the clinic, the social worker, the counselor—from whatever sources are maintained by the program staff. These sources will be described at length in chapter 6. Why, then, would one include a large section in the survey on the utilization of services? Since both the numerator and denominator of the survey data is restricted to those in school on the day of the survey (unfortunately, with high rates of absenteeism, that can represent under 80 percent of the student body), of what use is the self-report of the respondents on the services they used, when a more accurate count can be found in the service records themselves?

The answer is that only in the aggregate survey data do we have the opportunity to understand *who used* and *who did not use* the services. Only in the aggregate survey data can we link the respondents' self-reported utilization of specific services to their knowledge, attitudes, and behaviors, and even to their own reported reasons for use and non-use of the program's facilities. Analyzing the data in this manner, we can develop a great deal of information vital to the upgrading or evaluation of an intervention; for example, in a pregnancy prevention program, what proportion of those who did *not* use the contraceptive services were not using them because they were not sexually active? Similarly, evaluators of an intervention to prevent substance abuse might want to know whether those who do not use its services are smokers, drinkers, drug users; whether or not they use other prevention programs; whether they can be described by any other characteristics reported in the questionnaire.

The implications of this use of the survey data for the selection of variables to include in the study is already addressed (see pages 61–63). The data add immensely to the richness of our understanding because they give us as complete a picture of those who *do not* use a program as they do of those who *do*. This is a dimension of evaluation which is never achieved by studies that must rely on information, however detailed, on a program's clients alone—for example, on records of the self-selected group of patients who walked through a clinic's doors.

What is interesting about these variables in the analysis phase is their use, alternatively, as both independent and dependent variables. When trying to determine who uses and who does not use certain services, for example, utilization variables may be treated as *outcomes*. Given that a girl is at or ahead of grade level, started sex at fifteen or older, holds strong feelings against adolescent childbearing, and has discussed contraception with her boyfriend, is she more or less likely to use the clinic? Given that a boy has friends who use drugs, wants to go to college, has experimented with several substances, is he more or less likely to have used the counseling services a program provides?

Alternatively, the same variables can be seen as *independent variables*, with reported recent behaviors serving as the outcomes. Given that a respondent attended the clinic, was she more or less likely to use contraception at last coitus? Given that a respondent spoke to a counselor, was he more or less likely to smoke marijuana in the last four weeks?

The utilization variables can be used in a third way as well; they can serve as *intervening variables*, telling us whether, given certain background characteristics, use or non-use of the program had more or less impact. Thus, did a girl's discussion with her partner about contraception lead to attendance/nonattendance at rap sessions, and in turn did that increase or decrease her chance of considering contraception *now*? Was it on those who had or those who had not previously thought of contraception that program contact had the most effect?

As these several examples should suggest, the time frame to which the variables in the questionnaire apply becomes critical when using them in the analysis. What happened *after* the program opened can only be ascertained for a few time-related variables, and what *predated* the program may not be available except for some background characteristics which are unlikely to be affected by the program at all. If change in any behavioral variables is to be related to program *exposure,* dates of those behaviors must be identified; if they are to be related to program *utilization,* dates of that utilization must be available as well.

Finally, a serious attempt must be made to understand selection processes among those who make use of program components. Two examples should suffice: (1) If the baseline suggests that those who used professional contraceptive facilities in the absence of the special intervention were young women who reported the highest frequencies of coitus in the last month, it should not be surprising if the same is the case when the new program is in place. If one were to discover that attendance at the program facility was related to high frequencies of coitus, that would not imply that the program causes more frequent sex. It would merely suggest that those with frequent exposure to coitus were more likely to attend contraceptive clinics. (2) If absenteeism is higher among students enrolled in a comprehensive clinic than among those who are not enrolled, that does not tell us that health clinics cause absenteeism. It may imply that parents of the least healthy students were more likely to return the consent form to enroll their children as patients. Only if we know their levels of absenteeism before enrollment and after, or know enough about their health to make adequate comparisons with the baseline data, can we come to conclusions on the effects of the clinic itself.

Interpreting "Soft" Data

When dealing with areas as sensitive as these, there is always question as to the reliability of the data. The willingness of young men and women to answer honestly, their ability to understand the language, and the seriousness with which they undertake the task can all affect the accuracy of their response. These are legitimate areas for concern, but the evidence from countless surveys is that data from school questionnaires are generally of surprisingly good quality. How can one tell? What caveats are there when interpreting questionnaires replete with retrospective dates, self-reported attitudes and perceptions, and behaviors the young respondents might well have wished to hide?

First of all, there will be a few "completed" questionnaires that are clearly useless—but probably not very many. Young people are usually curious about the questionnaire; many are at an altruistic age which makes them respond when they believe that honest answers can help their peers. Very few appear to write off the survey process as a joke. A few exceptions will be obvious the moment the questionnaires are examined because they will contain comments in the margin, nonsense answers, multiple responses to variables that require only one answer—all aberrations that signal that the entire questionnaire must be set aside. We tabulated these as we did refusals, and all together they totaled a very small percentage. Other researchers report similar encouraging results.

There is some evidence that questions in even such sensitive areas as pregnancy are generally answered honestly. Occasionally, there are individual replies that must be considered "out of range" even in an otherwise responsible questionnaire: age four for first intercourse, 100 partners last month, and the like. A researcher will have to look at all distributions and make some rational decisions about which to allow and which to omit from the summary data. Another way of handling such outliers is to include them in broad groupings such as "low, medium, and high." Our experience and that of others suggests that the numbers of aberrational replies should be few.

Internal consistency is a good check on the reliability of the data as well. As described in appendix D, crosstabulations that expose inconsistencies are an important part of the data cleaning process.

The validity of the data can also be confirmed with reference to outside information; vital records can give a bench mark against which to confirm pregnancy data, even when the students do not necessarily come from specified census tracts. Clearly, there are many variables that cannot be checked against any outside information; indeed, that is why we need to collect them in these aggregate data in the first place! Nonetheless, a few of these internal and external verification procedures may add greatly to one's confidence in the reliability and validity of the data, and permit one to utilize the information to the full.

The best advice, however, is caution in the interpretation of the results. Small differences may be real in the data, even statistically significant, but unless there is consistency to the trend, or some similarity between the effects observed in related variables, it may not be possible to make a case for real, substantive change. Conversely, differences that appear of some importance may not achieve statistical importance because of the small size of the subgroup affected. Despite all the textbook rules, and despite the rigorous demands of evaluation, it is ultimately personal style and professional expertise that determine the usefulness of the final interpretation.

The logic of the relationships one observes must carry a great deal of weight. That is one reason that repeating surveys at several time periods adds to the strength of the study. Pregnancy, for example, changed in logical ways over time in the Hopkins study, adding greatly to our confidence. Abortion rates came down before birth rates in the program schools. A slowed increase preceded a decrease in pregnancies and was followed, after longer program exposure, by an even larger decrease. Rational relationships lend a good deal of confidence to our interpretation of the results.

Results can be statistically significant but still trivial; for example, even statistically significant changes in knowledge in two grades may mean little if four other grades show no change at all. But beyond the scientific judgement with respect to the importance of a finding, there is another dimension: its social importance. That is where the experience of the research team comes into play. If the two grades were the youngest grades, *and* if in every knowledge area explored the same relationships obtained, a significant change in only two grades could tell us something very important about the age-related impact of our program. The finding would no longer be trivial.

Other researchers will have their own styles and their own philosophies of interpretation. We tend to permit broad use of the materials the young people give us, but to exercise meticulous care in the coding, editing, and cleaning processes, and extreme caution in reporting the results. Major outcome measures need to show consistent change, change that can be observed even when different methods of analysis are used, before we are willing to claim that the evaluation demonstrates significant program effects.

6
Auxiliary Sources of Data

The basic source of data for program evaluation is the school questionnaire described in chapter 4, because it yields information on the entire student body regardless of services sought. However, other data can be collected from the program schools or from other sources to answer specific questions which cannot be examined using the schoolwide questionnaire. These data may include (1) detailed records completed for the students who enroll in the programs' clinics or services, (2) daily logs filled out by the service providers to record all student contacts and the nature of each contact, and (3) public access information on students and classroom counts provided by the school system. In some cities, the health department can provide birth or other relevant information that assists in evaluation as well. In addition, persons with one or another type of contact with the program can be surveyed; in the current program, for instance, a teacher questionnaire and a parent questionnaire were administered. The major difference between these types of data and the schoolwide questionnaire data is that most of these data can be identified by individual, making it possible to perform longitudinal analysis on the information collected, which cannot be done with aggregate, anonymous data. (In those evaluations in which survey data are not anonymous, no such difference exists.) Each program will, no doubt, have some of these types of data available, using staff records, public access records, or encounter records on subsets of the school population who make use of individual components of the program's offerings.

Most detailed in the current example are the clinic records, which can be designed to yield a large quantity of research material. Even in the absence of "basic" research, these records can be used on the simple level of "counting" when performing the evaluation. How many students use the clinic, how many boys/girls, how many medical enrollees, and so on—all these pieces of information can be gleaned from them. Similar counts can be estimated from the follow-up school questionnaires as well, if one is willing to rely on self-report. However, much more complete and accurate counts can be obtained from clinic records if they are properly maintained. The level of agreement between self-report and clinic records, in turn, yields an estimate of the validity of the student questionnaires.

The types of data collection described in this chapter may or may not be necessary to each evaluation, or may be of interest in truncated form. Judgments will have to be made in each project as to the level of detail and accuracy required, and the cost-effectiveness of maintaining and computerizing clinic and other personal records relative to the use that will, potentially, be made of them.

Clinic Records

Whatever the eligibility requirements or record requirements of a given school-linked program, they must both be rigorously defined if evaluation is contemplated. The records described here relate to the structure of the program for which they were designed, but can be adapted to other clinical initiatives and models as well. What is important is that eligibility be specified and codified and that records be designed in advance of program initiation.

In the project described here, all students from the two program schools, males and females alike, were eligible to get services at the program clinic for as long as they remained students at either program school. Thus, the numbers of students enrolled in the schools become the denominators for estimating the proportions served. Without defined eligibility, no such estimates can be made, and a basic measure of program achievement would be lacking.

As in any medical facility, records are filled out by providers when they see students in the program clinic, and these records become part of the students' charts. However, in a research project, providers must be required to fill out the forms *completely*, under guidance provided by the researchers. Some of this guidance can be in the form of ongoing consultation, and some involves the actual design of the instruments, as will be described. Most of the types of records detailed here have equivalent forms for clinics other than reproductive health facilities. We will indicate which records were included primarily for research, but even those basic to clinic operation must be designed with the research objective in mind.

Registration Forms

At an enrollment visit, an initial registration form, with basic information about the student, should be filled out by the registrar or some staff member who uniformly performs this task. (Some protocols may involve completing these forms on all students, without awaiting such a visit.) This information should include such information as the date of visit, the school identification

(ID) number (or whatever number will be used for this purpose), name, phone number, address, present school and class, date of entering a program school, date of birth, age, and sex. In the Hopkins program, it also included whether the visit was to be kept confidential, whether the enrollee had ever been to another clinic to get birth control (in other programs, this question can deal with the key offerings of the specific initiative), and whether and how many times the enrollee had visited the program clinic before registering.

Some of the previously mentioned variables need explanation; the first is the school ID number. All the clinic records about any one enrollee are usually kept in his or her chart, which, in most clinics, is identified and filed by name. Therefore, a numbering system is needed to identify patients for research without the use of names. Either for confidentiality, or because names are not always unique identifiers, numbers are required. One can assign each enrollee a clinic identification number at registration, but it is often simpler to use the school identification number. In a school system, each student is generally assigned a number when he or she enters the system for the first time; that number is retained until graduation or termination for some other reason. The advantages of this number for research are numerous: (1) It already exists and therefore is easy to adopt; (2) it is unique and allows all individual students to be identified whether or not they utilize any of the program's services; (3) it permits the research design to link the clinic data with other data collected. Although the school system's number may be longer than needed to identify each clinic enrollee uniquely, this disadvantage is outweighed by the many advantages of using an existing numerical code.

Students should also be asked the date on which they first entered a program school, in order to permit measurement of the duration of each student's exposure to the program before enrolling in the clinic or utilizing its services in other ways. At every visit, enrollees should be asked if there are any changes in address, phone, school, or class. Such changes can be noted on the registration form, and are useful primarily for getting in touch with the student; they are rarely used for research purposes.

Just as eligibility requirements must be carefully defined, so must "enrollment." In the present case, a student became a clinic enrollee when he or she registered at the clinic for the first time to get one of several specific services. In other programs, the definition of enrollment may be different: merely entering the clinic may be considered enrollment by one program; at the other extreme, another program may not wish to count students as enrolled unless they register for one specific service. Whatever the definition, "enrollment," to be counted, must be clearly specified.

Next, basic services must be specified. In the program described here, basic services included contraception, pregnancy tests, medical consultation (related to contraception or not so related, for example, sexually transmitted disease testing), individual counseling, and individual education, which included training of "peer resource" students. These services were designated in the record as "presenting reasons," and each visit was assigned such a reason by the provider. The assignment was based on the student's description of why he or she had come to the clinic. (This was not necessarily the reason the provider told the student to come, nor was it necessarily the sole service received, but it served a useful purpose in researching the motivation of students who sought out clinic services.) Similarly, in any clinic, the services that form the core of the program's offerings should be identified. Only in that way is it possible to describe clinic use as a function of *why the patient or client sought service* (rather than of what he or she *received* after medical or social evaluation.)

Finally, a grid sheet was also begun by the registrar at the first enrollment visit to record the date of each visit, and to list which forms had been filled out. This information was used to assign each visit a number and to identify the forms that had to be coded. It became a valuable research tool.

Consent Forms

At the time of the initial contact with the registrar, each student was requested to sign a consent form that covered services, confidentiality, the voluntary nature of the enrollee's participation, and the use of the clinic information for research purposes. Another consent form was filled out each time the clinic enrollee received a new type of contraceptive method. Although the consent is primarily for service reasons, maintenance of these forms is of major importance if any research is to be carried out using patient records. The records include personal identification, and must only be used for research if the patient has been so informed. The patient can be told that names will be removed when the data are used for research, if that is, indeed, the case. There is rarely any objection to the form when it is simply written and clearly explained by a sympathetic and supportive member of the staff. Permission can be given on the *same* form as the patient's medical consent or on a *separate* consent form, but in either case, researchers should be responsible for checking the consent forms before they are put in use, to be certain that their utilization of the data is covered. The procedure for refusing permission to use the forms for research, and for noting that refusal, should be clearly stated to each patient, and recorded as part of any protocol.

Medical Records

When an enrollee saw a medical provider to receive a medical service or to get contraception, a *medical visit form* was filled out. The form included items to record parity and the results of lab tests and physical exams. It permitted the provider to record the nature of the medical complaint, if any; a brief menstrual history, the contraceptive method in current use and that which was given during the visit; the provider's impression of the patient's general physical health; the date of the next scheduled appointment; and whether follow-up of an acute problem was indicated. Once again, date, name, ID number, and presenting reason were also recorded.

In addition, there was a *medical history form* that was filled out only for females at the first physical examination and at each annual examination thereafter. Information was collected about menstrual, sexual, contraceptive, pregnancy, and family medical histories, the patient's smoking status, chronic and acute conditions, and hospitalizations.

Pregnancy tests were performed at the clinic and a separate record was maintained of all tests and their outcomes. These could be used to flag tests in the individual records until they were computerized. In clinics that do not computerize all records, such independent lists of specific services can be the basis of research counts. They need to be carefully maintained.

Social Records

Most females had a social-psychological assessment by one of the program social workers. This assessment was updated yearly. The information collected included who referred the student to the clinic, who accompanied her there, whether her family knew she was there, sources of family income, whether the student was presently working, household structure, the age of the patient's mother and of her oldest child (allowing computation of the mother's age at first birth), and the patient's sexual, contraceptive, and pregnancy history.

Social workers and counselors often collect information in the form of discursive "notes"; these are almost impossible to code without enormous expense. Even if one were to expend the time and funds, the data are not very useful because the notations are not parallel from one record to another. It is therefore important to consult with the counseling staff and to design forms that capture those dimensions of the clients' communications—and the social workers' assessments—that will be valuable to researcher and counselor alike. If tapped before the forms are printed, the researcher's expertise and knowledge of prior literature in the field can supplement the social worker's perceptions, and the social worker's experience can enlarge the scope of the study. Time invested in a creative interchange *while forms are still in the design phase* can result in forms that preserve useful information that might otherwise be lost.

The "Non-Form" Form

Finally, there was a catchall form available to note a visit that did not require one of the preceding forms. In our case, it was most frequently used to record the distribution of condoms and foam, to indicate when the patient received education and counseling, and/or when the social worker met with the clinic patient without completing a social-psychological assessment. A clinic that is not involved in a research protocol may not feel the need of such a back-up form, but it is generally important to document all program contacts. It is essential to do so in a research situation because dates of visits might not otherwise be backed up by a "paper trail"—a frustrating problem when records are systematized for future study.

Maintaining Records for Research

Ensuring Record Quality

Most of the preceding information would have been collected with or without a research project, since a great deal of it is covered by standard operating procedure in a responsible reproductive health clinic. However, providers are generally not as meticulous about filling in all the information on a record as researchers would wish them to be. They frequently fail to distinguish between missing information which was not collected because it was inapplicable, and that which was not collected for some other, perhaps significant, reason. When medical personnel—the worst offenders—enter a dash in a space, it can mean "We did not perform this test" or "The results were normal" or "The results have not come in yet" or simply "I do not know." Confusing these options is not acceptable practice for the researcher. For evaluators, certain information *always* needs to be recorded; it must be recorded using only established codes, and in its absence, it is necessary to include the reasons for which it is omitted from the record. Researchers should work with providers to design intake forms that are clear to read, easy to fill in, and unequivocal to code. One excellent device to help ensure complete data is to put an asterisk next to all items that are to be coded, as a reminder that these items require special attention. This method of "flagging" specific variables is useful to the busy provider and serves the researcher well. It is strongly recommended to those who seek to use clinic records for research purposes.

Data for Research Only

It may be that some information is collected solely for research purposes. That is a more unusual situation, which will probably be encountered only in programs that share service and academic objectives, and hence are funded to permit the investment of staff time in the collection of research data. The fact that these data are primarily research tools, however, need not suggest that they are of no value to the service program if used creatively. In fact, the integration of information collection with any aspect of a service program may be a measure of the excellence of the "marriage" of research and service.

One example may suffice: There was, in the index program, one fairly complex set of information collected by the social workers solely for research. This was a month-by-month sexual history calendar filled out at the time of the first social-psychological assessment. The calendar was updated (1) at an annual visit, (2) when there was a change in contraceptive method, and (3) at an exit interview. On a calendar grid, the box in the first row, first column, represented the first month and year of the individual's sexual calendar, the date of her first coital experience. The other eleven columns in the first row were for the next eleven months. Row two started the next twelve months, and so on, up to the month and year of the present clinic contact. Detailed information was recorded for each month in which the respondent had sexual intercourse at least once, including what contraceptive method she used, the number of times she had sex, and with which partner she had sex. In addition, the conception, gestation, and outcome of each pregnancy were recorded at the appropriate dates. Boxes representing months in which the respondent did not have intercourse were crosshatched.

Clearly, this information goes further than would ordinarily have been required in a social worker's interview, but it can readily be seen that many of the areas probed would be valuable in understanding the needs of the patient. Skillful counselors can use the data collection process to stimulate open communication, rather than as an extraneous interruption to the counseling process. The same might be true in other types of programs where obtaining histories of substance use, employment, schooling, family structure, and so on, might be included in the research agenda. Severe limits must be imposed by the service staff on such data collection in the interests of time, patient flow, and "overload" on the counseling relationship, but a creative balance between research and service should allow room for the recording of information that might contribute some interesting new insights.

Routinizing Service Protocols for Research

At times, the program staff may be asked to put defined parameters on its procedures purely for research purposes. In this case, they may be carrying out a service that is a necessary part of their operation, but doing so in a way that permits the researchers to count or to identify its recipients. For example, if counts were needed of the numbers of students to see a particular film strip, the educator might be asked to take a specified number of students into each session, or to record the number present and close the door, letting no one stroll in uncounted in the course of the session.

At other times, protocols themselves may be defined with the research objective in mind. This means that a routine procedure must be designed, and must be adhered to, by the program staff. For example, we were interested in testing how many reminders, and of what kind, it would take in a school setting to bring female patients back for their annual visits. A plan was worked out with the providers to specify what written and personal reminders would be used, to schedule them at regular and established intervals, and to record them for each patient when she was due for her visit. This information was coded for special study. The protocols did not have an adverse effect on the service, although they did require a formal organization of the follow-up procedure; they yielded useful results which could not have been obtained in the absence of the research design. In addition, when students did return for annual visits, they filled out anonymous questionnaires including some basic background/demographic variables, contraceptive and pregnancy knowledge, contraceptive and pregnancy behavior, reasons for which the patient came to the clinic, and services received. Once again, routinizing the data collection made it useful to providers and researchers alike.

Informal Research Protocols

Still another variation is the service procedure that is part of the clinic protocol, and incidentally yields informal information that is of value to the research and service staff. For example, a special initiative adopted by the educators as an experiment may have to be monitored on a temporary basis to assess its acceptance by the students. A routine procedure may have to be tested to see if it has the desired effect. Short time periods can be designated to ask certain questions of every student, or to count the students who utilize a service. A few weeks may be long enough for these informal checks, but care must be taken to choose a time slot that is as close to normal operation as possible (for example, not during vacation, exam week, or stormy weather). The most valuable use of these tests is in what is described in chapter 1 as formative or process evaluation; the information is fed back into the program to improve its design and service.

Other informal research can use a clinic routine to answer important issues related to our understanding of the patient population. A central issue, the need for confidentiality of clinic service, was addressed in the current program in the following way: At the enrollment visit, students were asked if it was all right to contact them at home and/or if their mothers knew they were coming to the clinic for services. If they answered "no," the registrar stamped "CONFIDENTIAL" in large red capital letters on the folders of their charts while they were watching. It made it clear and visible that the clinic meant to abide by their requests. In their personal contacts with the patients, staff stressed the importance of family communication, although they did not do so in the context of this decision. At every subsequent visit, students were asked the same question. If the answer changed from no to yes, "CONFIDENTIAL" was scratched out and the date noted. We then had a record of how many enrollees discussed the clinic visit with their mothers initially, and how many did so after their first visits. This measure of confidentiality yields data that is soft, at best. Since the question was an oral one, it may not always have been asked in exactly the same way; what it meant from enrollee to enrollee and visit to visit may, therefore, have been different. However, as a means of assessing the importance of confidentiality to the population as a whole, or estimating the general impact of the program's emphasis on communication, it is nonetheless useful.

Similar creative means of furthering a program's objectives, and maintaining counts of the effectiveness of its initiatives, can add to the richness of the evaluation. Initiatives need not be in place from the outset of the program to be examined in this way; as long as dates are recorded and patient visits can be counted by date, a denominator for an experimental intervention can be calculated, and an informal estimate made of the impact of each new idea.

Termination Dates

One other piece of information important for research is the date the student is no longer eligible to receive services. In the program described here, students were eligible to receive services as long as they were students in either program school, which is probably the case in many school-based initiatives. Some programs may serve an entire community; in that case, eligibility numbers would be hard to estimate, and there may be no "termination" date at all. Generally, however, eligibility for a school-based initiative terminates when enrollment does, even if that termination occurs in the course of the school year. With all the movement into and out of schools, whether or not the clinic is located in the school, it may be difficult to keep track of every student. One is dependent on information in the clinic charts, or on the lists the school system makes available, to determine when an individual's program eligibility terminates. This information is relevant because a student who is only eligible for two months after his or her first visit probably differs in clinic utilization from a student who has two more years available in which to use the clinic. Thus, to know whether the behavior observed was reflective of clinic use patterns or was related only to the length of eligibility, termination information must be available. Those who run school-linked clinics might well make an effort to have a good system set up in advance to obtain and maintain this information. Doing so can also simplify the follow-up procedures they develop as a part of the service component.

Other Records and Data

Staff Log Records

The single most exhaustive task carried out by the staff for research purposes was recording their day-to-day activities. Time allocation is a process well known to many professionals, but unusual in the social service setting. In this case, every day, the four major service providers—the two social workers and the two nurses—filled out log records. On these forms they listed the names of the students with whom they had contact that day and noted what services they rendered them both in school and in the clinic. These records can be used to estimate the costs of the program's components when used in conjunction with estimates of the time each staff member spends rendering each type of service, and the costs of the allocated time. Along with the clinic data, they can also describe a student's total experience in, or utilization of, the program.

A more complete history was obtained by linking these data, using the school identification number, with data from the school system. The school system created computer tapes for each school for each of the three program years to give the researchers a complete record of all students who were in the schools during the course of the program. This information served two very useful purposes. The first was to assign background/demographic characteristics (for example, age, grade, curriculum, free lunch, zip code) to all the students so more could be known about them than whether they did or did not utilize any program services. The second was to enable us to calculate a denominator equal to the total number of eligible students, as described in chapter 3. Failing this, one would have had only limited ability to estimate the percentages of all students in the schools who received various services.

Using this entire log/clinic data set, as large and varied as it is, a wide range of issues can be examined, including: numbers of student contacts by provider and by age and gender of students, program costs for services and individuals, the cost-effectiveness of the program as a whole and in its separate components, patterns of use of the school and clinic services, and the relationship between those patterns and the adoption of contraception.

Research costs for a large, combined data set of this kind are high, as is the time allocation required to enter and systematize it. If the data are not to be used for a detailed cost-effectiveness analysis or for basic research, should they be collected? The answer is probably yes, but only on a selective basis. A few months invested in monitoring staff time allocations could be extremely valuable. Overuse or underuse of staff in certain locations or for specified tasks can be pinpointed. A study of the logs could tell the program's administrators a great deal about the utilization of components of service by the target population. Taken in combination with the anonymous, aggregate data on program utilization, some judgements can be made about the success of the program in allocating appropriate amounts of time to the services the students find most useful, and might even lead to a reappraisal of staff assignments. In combination with cost data, informal estimates of cost-effectiveness can be made, which can be of importance for management and refunding even if a formal analysis is beyond the scope of the research. But unless a long-term investment in cost analysis or basic research is contemplated, maintaining such records for prolonged periods will not pay.

Class Records

For each round of the questionnaire, the schools provided listings of the number of male and female students enrolled in each classroom. Teachers supplemented this information by indicating how many students of each sex were present on the day the questionnaire was administered and how many of them refused to take the survey. These numbers were used for two purposes. First, they determined the number of questionnaires of each type to deliver to each classroom. Second, they yielded the denominators for calculating coverage rates and response rates. Coverage rates were calculated by dividing the number of usable questionnaires by the number of students *enrolled* in the school at the time of the survey. Response rates were calculated by dividing the number of usable questionnaires by the number of students *present* in the school on the day of the survey. The complement of the response rate is the refusal rate.

Birth Records

There have been some attempts to utilize birth records as a measure of school birth rates, especially in programs in which it is impossible to collect baseline data. The researchers request from the school system the enrollment rolls for several years before the program was in place, and for several years during the program. They compile lists of all of the students by name, grade, and years of attendance. These lists are forwarded to the health department, which checks them against birth records. After entering information on all births appearing in the official records, including dates of births, the names are removed and the lists are returned to the researchers. It is then possible for the researchers to determine which young women were in the schools at their dates of conception (by subtracting nine months) and thus to determine a birth rate for the school both before and after the program. Researchers who have used this method report that it probably yields valid information in that they believe most of the births are captured in this way. However, they report that there is a good deal of variation year to year, which makes it difficult to ascertain whether there is a true trend, even when the fluctuations are rather large. (There is always the possibility that people exposed to the program have already dropped out of the school at the time they conceived; one could include them if "exposure" to the program were under study rather than "access" to the program clinic, but to the best of our knowledge that has not been done.) One possible source of error would be young women who do not deliver in the same jurisdiction, but the assumption has to be made that they do not contribute a significant portion of births.

It is our hope that health departments throughout the nation could be convinced to include school of attendance at the time of conception in birth certificates for all women eighteen years old and younger. If the concept of delivering services to young women within the school context is to be adequately tested in the future, such a simple addition to the birth record could contribute a great deal to the ease with which these data could be compiled. In the absence of such a notation, the method just described is a useful one, and a viable alternative to collecting the data by self-report alone. The most serious problem with this method is that it relates to childbirth only; if our interest is in pregnancy, the omission of information on abortion is a serious limitation.

Related Questionnaires

Most programs that deliver medical and social services to teens are many faceted, and present opportunities for the study of a wide range of associated services. The extent to which these supplemental areas should be explored, in view of the costs of adding them to the basic evaluation, should be carefully assessed. In the present program, two such facets of outreach presented interesting opportunities. One was an examination of whether and how the program affected the attitudes of the teachers, and whether and how these factors affected the outcome of the program. In a longer project, this kind of data could have answered the question: Can school services be designed utilizing the input of the teachers in the program schools? Would that add to program effectiveness? Another area of investigation involved a pilot program for parents of seventh graders, to improve communication between them and their children. Although neither of these aspects of the program were utilized in the final evaluation, we will discuss the questionnaires so that others interested in doing studies using these populations will benefit from these pilot endeavors. They illustrate the extent to which interlocking data sets can be useful, if care is exercised in matching the questions so they can be comparable one to the other.

Teacher questionnaires were administered anonymously, one time only, to teachers in each of the four schools included in the study. Teachers answered their questionnaires while the students were filling in theirs. Information collected included sex, marital status, race, and age of the teacher, and whether he or she had any children and, if so, the ages of the oldest and youngest children. A variety of questions from the student questionnaires were then asked of the teachers. These included attitudes to sexual intercourse, responsibility for contraception, and what a girl should do if she gets pregnant by a boy she does not love; best ages for sex, marriage, and being a parent; perception of method efficacy; under what circumstances it is all right for a woman to have an abortion; the ten questions about contraceptive knowledge, pregnancy risk, and abortion; and the four questions about the need for parents' consent to get reproductive health services (see chapter 4). Teachers were also asked questions about sex education in school; in particular, they were asked whether it should be offered in school and what topics it should cover. They were asked how a teacher should handle questions about conception and who were the most appropriate persons to help a high school youngster with questions about having sex, contraception, abortion, pregnancy and parenting, and using drugs. The teachers were also asked how comfortable they were talking to students about sexual matters and whether they would like further training to do so. These questions could be useful in determining to what extent teacher input might be valuable in designing in-school programs, and/or to what extent faculty may be a part of the problem rather than a part of the solution.

The initial objective of the seventh-grade parents' project was to interview the mother of each seventh-grade child in the program school, the index child, in the first year of the program. This was accomplished, and, although these interviewer-administered questionnaires are not well tested, they tap an important dimension of adolescent services. The first set of questions related to the background of the child and the parents, including current household structure, whether the parent works, and source of family income. Again, questions from the student questionnaires were utilized: perception of method efficacy; attitudes towards having sex and contraceptive responsibility; and knowledge about pregnancy risk and contraception. Parents were asked their beliefs about the best time for them to talk to children about having sex; who is the best person to tell children about sex; what subjects are "okay" to teach children in school; and discussions they, the parents, have had with the index child about puberty, sex, contraception, teen parenting, pregnancy risk, VD, and substance abuse. They were asked for whom teenage parenthood causes problems; whether or not they would like it if the index child did not graduate from high school, had sex, and got pregnant (or got a girl pregnant); and whether the index child had had sex and had had (or had fathered) a baby. They were asked other questions about the child relating to his or her friends, activities in which the child participates when not in school, and whether or not the parent also participates. The responsibilities the child has in the home are explored, as is the time the child has to be home at night, and how often the parent is home when the child returns home from school. Parents also were asked a series of questions about their experiences: whether as teens they had talked to their parents about sex, contraception, pregnancy, and substance abuse; what contraceptive methods they had ever used and the regularity with which birth control is currently used; females were asked about their first pregnancy outcomes, and their ages at the time of those outcomes. Finally, respondents were asked if they were interested in participating in community workshops, and if yes, what times and places were preferable.

As basic research, the parent and student questionnaires were linked by date of birth of the seventh grader and other information (maintaining careful procedures to guarantee anonymity of the aggregate data for which anonymity had been promised) to look at parent/child communication. It was found that there is not always agreement between the two on these variables. This leads to a general problem which must be understood when launching companion studies of this kind: To what extent do such contradictory responses reflect problems in the data, and to what extent does disagreement represent an important finding in its own right? If the original data are as reliable and valid as one hopes they are, the contradictions may tell us something substantive and useful. However, when dealing with subjective variables, or retrospective variables recollected after long intervals, extreme caution needs to be exercised in interpreting these data. That need not prohibit their collection, because the insights which may be gained into the attitudes, the knowledge, and even the behaviors of the adults who interface with adolescents may be useful even if the data are insufficiently robust to form the basis for independent research.

These two ancillary surveys are suggestive of the range of related material that could contribute to our understanding of school-linked initiatives. One could envision similar attempts to collect data from community leaders, from youth service agencies, or from medical providers serving a neighborhood, town, or district in which school programs are located. Although such studies might enrich our knowledge, they are generally not focal to the evaluation. In particular situations one might foresee, however, they could be crucial to the study, and one would hope the researchers were in close enough contact to know when that might be the case. For example, if there are crosscurrents in the community that are not well understood, surveys might be used to pinpoint sources of potential support or opposition, and thus could help explain the success or failure of the larger program.

Process Evaluation: How Did It Work?

In addition to these data sources, one of the often missing links in program evaluation is a narrative description of what the program was all about. Process evaluation entails a sense of what went on—a qualitative account of the content of the services, the performance of the staff, the philosophy of the planners, and the reactions of the participants. It includes not only what was meant to happen but what actually did occur, including barriers to effective service and unexpected success. (There is a more detailed description of process evaluation in chapter 1.)

The log data previously described give a *count* of a wide range of services; the various services can be grouped to yield a manageable number of service components to describe in some detail. Which individual services become important enough to highlight should emerge in the early period of the program. The task of the evaluators will be greatly simplified if, with a little foresight, these services are identified in time to include the same groupings in the utilization questions of the follow-up surveys. In that way, researchers can link students' self-reported use of and attitudes toward these services with the staff's descriptions of the same program components. In turn, the costs of the same components can be established. If services are differently grouped and classified in each data set, it is hard to sort them out at a later date.

In large measure, process evaluation is a task for the program staff, who may need to be coaxed into putting on paper details of their day-to-day activities. Evaluators may wish to supplement the accounts obtained from staff with materials from student surveys, focus groups, exit interviews, or client satisfaction forms. Any of a number of ways to collect clients' input can be devised. What is important is to put flesh on the skeletal descriptions of program models which are often all that is available to the provider who would like to replicate a successful intervention. The individuality and personal inprint of program staff is, of course, hard to transfer, but the more we can recall and communicate of the flavor of a program that works, the more we will contribute to the larger field.

Last Words

Wen the time is ripe, when a field is exploring new frontiers, the impact of good evaluation can be dramatic. It can spur providers to replicate and create; it can stir legislators out of their lethargies of fear; it can reach professionals at every level of public and private service. This makes the endeavor worth all the effort we have described.

The initial evaluation based on our methodology (originally published in *Family Planning Perspectives*) can be found in appendix A. This is only one report out of the many that can flow from the techniques we have suggested. Basic research, component analysis, cost-effectiveness studies— all utilize the same data sets. Individual cohorts can be followed, starting when they enter the school and tracking them through their years of exposure. Behavioral histories before and after the program can be analyzed in order to understand its impact. The methods we propose can be used to measure the effects not only of pregnancy prevention programs but of comprehensive health initiatives, alcohol clinics, drug prevention programs, smoking cessation and weight control initiatives, and school enrichment programs. Once the extensive data are in hand, they can serve many creative purposes in program development and in the formation of public policy.

Use of the School Base for Evaluation

The research format we present can be used for whatever programs have a service and/or an educational or counseling component; it can be used whenever there is good reason to believe that knowledge, attitudes, or behaviors, or any combination of those dimensions, might change. It can be used for whatever programs define the school as a population in which that change might best be observed.

We suggested in the introduction that schools might increasingly become the focus of research—a natural unit within which programs for adolescents are assessed. Does this imply that services themselves will necessarily be centered within school walls? Must a school be the locus of a program in order to be the focus of the research design? Not necessarily; the model on which this book is based should make it clear that a program can be planned in concert with a school, that it can make a powerful difference to a student body, provide services, and change essential patterns of behavior—without delivering its medical services within the school setting. It is appropriate therefore to use the research design proposed here whenever there is good reason to believe a particular school is being reached by a community program, even if all its services are not physically rendered within the school itself.

This is not to say that services whose relationships with local schools are merely casual, or accidentally contiguous, are likely candidates; the research model is too exhaustive, the investment of time and funds too great, to embark upon unless there is some reason to believe the school connection is a real one. But one can envision a wide range of situations in which the research model can be used. For example:

1. A community has a health/drug/pregnancy prevention program based in a high-risk area with little obvious impact on the nearby schools. The baseline survey we propose is administered and confirms both the high level of need and the low level of program utilization that were hypothesized. An outreach staff is placed in the local schools each day to bring the educational component of the program into the school setting, to become familiar with and to the student body, to take histories, counsel, teach, and/or assist students to get to the facility—whatever roles are appropriate to the service initiative. Repeat surveys, logs at the school and other program sites, and the other techniques proposed here are used to measure the impact of that minimal additional investment in a strong outreach component, without moving the facility, itself, into the school.

2. A school-based clinical initiative is proposed for a middle, junior, and/or senior high. The community has reservations about the provision of certain services. A survey is used as a needs assessment tool, at one and the same time as it provides the baseline against which progress can be measured. Its results can also be used as an educational device; working with a community board and/or with the entire school family, its information can be helpful in bringing about consensus on the services that should be offered.

3. As in the model described in these pages, a proposed clinic is physically located outside the school in order to increase its availability to more than one school; to reduce costs accordingly—as one medical facility serves two or more schools; to permit the program to serve dropouts and absentees; and to minimize political pressures on its selection of services. Nonetheless, its strong in-school component makes it logical to measure impact on students in that target setting.

Similarly, programs with a larger proportion of their effort focused in the community, on groups other than those of school age, may still be validly assessed for their impact on community schools. In fact, one of the best ways to establish the value of family-focused initiatives may be by assessing their impact on young people in their formative school years. In any setting where a school is a part of a community, school-based evaluation could be a logical choice.

It should be clear, then, that school-based evaluation does not imply the existence of a "school-based clinic." As programs are tested, if successful models are identified and diffused, it is important that no single stereotype be imposed; no single design will serve every neighborhood well. In the face of budgetary cuts, political controversy, and serious rethinking of our national commitment to education, the field of adolescent services requires all the creativity and energy it can get, backed up by solid, objective research. In the present climate, the community may more and more often become the focus of program development and planning, and the center from which local initiatives grow. This need not imply a lesser role for the school, but perhaps a larger one, because any program that serves a community well, and that includes components of interest to teenage boys and girls, should have components within the school setting as a major point of contact with that age group. Alternatively, if a program has an impact on families that include youngsters of school age, the impact should be observable within the school context. Evaluation such as that we describe here clearly has a more important role than the assessment of school-based clinics alone.

Evaluation of Ongoing Programs

The evaluation model presented here relies heavily on the opportunity to collect baseline data from the program sites *before* intervention programs are put into place. That is not always possible. Much that is said in these chapters does not apply when a program is already underway, because the ability to select nonequivalent controls, with the emphasis on change as the primary unit of measurement, and other fundamentals of our model, depend on the data collection we describe. There are some methods that can still be used, focusing on the entering grades (sixth or seventh in junior high schools, ninth or tenth in senior highs). If data are collected early in the fall in experimental and control schools, the program should not yet have an effect on the entering classes; in that case, the comparative levels of change over time between the two groups of schools can still be useful. However, while all is not lost, this is not an evaluation design one can recommend. The inability to pretest older students denies one baseline information on the levels of change to be expected in the program schools between younger and older grades. Without randomization of samples (practically impossible in a school situation) or pre-tests, non-equivalent control groups are of limited use. It is only the entry of new grades each year, presumably from schools that do not have the special program, that allows one to preserve some information that is in the nature of a pre-test for a subset of students. These are the only students who can be compared with the control school entrants, and among whom change over time can be observed, in association with specific numbers of years of program exposure. As long as one restricts analysis to these groups, one can follow them over time and achieve many of the same results.

Who Can Do It?

Providers and funders will probably wonder who can perform the kinds of evaluative research we describe. Does it require a major input from a separate research staff? Are there any portions of these protocols that, following the steps we outline, can be carried out by the program staff itself? We will run through various components of the research model presented here and make some assessment of the minimum staff input required to carry out the evaluation:

1. Designing intake/encounter forms should be a cooperative task. Although some input from those who will code and analyze them is extremely helpful, a program staff can create the forms with the help of a part-time consultant, and with attention to some of the hints we include in chapter 6.

2. Once the techniques we describe for studying particular, short-term components of service are mastered, providers can organize their own service components for study. They can set up their own designs for counting entrants into a specific program, assessing the amount of contact needed to bring them in, comparing two different protocols for obtaining the same result, and so on. With appropriate feedback mechanisms in place, these techniques can add an important dimension to program administration, and can be carried out largely by the service staff.

3. Staff logs can be kept for selected time periods, supervised by the program administrator. With some investment of time, these can be used to count contacts, determine the flow of clients through the program, and estimate time invested in each activity. Combining these findings with costs, the administrator should be able to generate a cost-effectiveness estimate accurate enough to utilize for funding or planning purposes.

4. When it comes to the schoolwide questionnaire, the essential evaluation tool, program staff are *not* the right persons to carry out the study. Their input is needed, first, to determine the outcomes they seek to achieve and, second, to be certain the right components of service are included in the final assessment tool. They are an excellent resource for the evaluators

for insights into the problems, attitudes, or idiom of their target populations. They can also have a large role in the survey's administration especially when rapport with their schools is established. They are not the right persons to operationalize the outcomes into survey variables in the completed survey instrument, nor to conduct the analysis and calculate the final results. This is both because they will rarely possess the skills to carry out the kinds of analyses which are required, and, perhaps more important, because doing so might damage the scientific credibility which is demanded of a program evaluation. Always important in any assessment report, objectivity is even more crucial when one is operating on the cutting edge of public policy.

Conclusion

The complexity of the evaluation process is a function, in part, of current perceptions of health interventions not merely as dependent on the professional *services* or the supply side, but on the attitudes, knowledge, and receptivity of the *clients*, the demand side of the health service equation. If we were merely measuring the shape of professional services on the one hand, and pregnancy rates, substance use rates, and so on on the other, the task would be demanding, but not as sophisticated as the assessment of those human and institutional characteristics that may mediate behavioral change. Those subtle and elusive characteristics are often what make a program succeed or fail; it is the task of the evaluator to ferret them out.

We suggested at the outset that evaluation of strong and creative programs might help move the field of adolescent pregnancy prevention into a new generation of service—the dissemination of successful models. So, too, evaluations that go a step further and tell us what *components* of a program work, or better yet *how* a program works, can make replication more efficient and even suggest patterns of intervention that extend into other areas of adolescent behavior. The spirit of experimentation and individuality, so vital to new initiatives, should not be threatened by this evaluation/replication process; rather, good evaluation should be able to capture the essence of the creative endeavor and make it accessible to those who would learn from it. In the absence of some tangible proof of program effects, other professionals tend either to reinvent interventions one could have predicted would not work or, worse, to dismiss successful initiatives as the unique contributions of individual personalities, and therefore as unreplicable flukes. In either case, information that could have advanced the field is lost, to the detriment of providers, funders, and above all teenagers themselves.

Programs bringing services to adolescents in a school setting, or in connection with a school-based program, are potentially controversial, because parents are usually not present when treatment is rendered. When these programs include or focus upon pregnancy prevention, the potential for controversy increases, even though the majority of parents are supportive of such interventions. There are critics of new initiatives, albeit a minority, who will attempt to discredit services by attacking the evaluation techniques that prove them efficacious. This is why we have recommended throughout that any adjustments necessary when handling the data be made in the direction of minimizing, rather than maximizing, positive program effects. Doing so will increase confidence in the programs and policies the findings suggest to those who would replicate their models, and at the same time will strengthen the evaluation when, for political reasons, their conclusions come under attack. It is incumbent on the researchers to be "purer than Caesar's wife" in their methods and procedures, not only to maintain their own scientific standards, but because they might otherwise do damage to their programs and, indeed, to the field.

On the other hand, the potential for making a substantial contribution to adolescent services is real. Community-based planning, school-linked initiatives, adolescent services—these are concepts that are current and vital. They await the demonstration that strong, effective models exist, and the scientific proof that they work. When providers and researchers, together, can make that case, the "dry" field of evaluation comes to life. It can become the backbone of good program design, and can bring a breath of sanity to the contentious world of public policy.

Appendix A
Evaluation of a Pregnancy Prevention Program for Urban Teenagers

Laurie S. Zabin
Marilyn B. Hirsch
Edward A. Smith
Rosalie Streett
Janet B. Hardy

I n this article, we report on a school-based program for the primary prevention of pregnancy among inner-city adolescents that was designed and administered by the staff of The Johns Hopkins School of Medicine's Department of Pediatrics and Department of Gynecology and Obstetrics. The project was carried out with the cooperation of the administrators of four schools in the Baltimore school system—two junior high schools and two senior high schools. The program provided the students attending one of the junior high schools and one of the senior high schools with sexuality and contraceptive education, individual and group counseling, and medical and contraceptive services over a period of almost three school years. Students in the remaining two schools received no such services, but provided baseline and end-of-project data, and serve as the control sample.

An evaluation component, designed to assess changes in the knowledge, attitudes and behavior of the school populations, was built into the project from the outset. The evaluation was based on aggregate data collected from the students through self-administered questionnaires. The surveys were administered in the two program schools at four different times: once before the program began (at the start of the school year), and again during the spring term of each of the following three years. At the two control schools, questionnaires were given to the students at the beginning and at the end of the experimental program period.

The questionnaires asked the students for detailed information on their knowledge, attitudes and behavior relative to sexual conduct, contraception,

Reprinted with permission from *Family Planning Perspectives*, Volume 8, Number 3 May/June 1986 and teenage pregnancy and parenthood. It asked them about communication with their parents and partners, their educational aspirations and a range of demographic and background variables. Students in the seventh and eighth grades received a slightly abbreviated series of questions.

Parents were notified of the survey in advance and were informed that their children could be withdrawn from the study if they wished. Only two parents from the four schools made that request.

The junior high school in which the pregnancy prevention program was introduced is a community school serving an all-black, inner-city population. The average socioeconomic status in the community is low, and a high proportion of the students attending the school live in high-rise public housing. Almost nine out of 10 of the students qualify for the school's free lunch program. The senior high school involved in the program serves as both a magnet and a community school. For this reason, the small ninth-grade class and subsets of students in grades 10–12 are of somewhat higher academic standing than the other students, and are drawn from the entire city, while the remaining students in those grades come from the same general area that feeds the junior high school. All the students are black, and almost three-quarters qualify for free lunches. At the baseline survey, 667 male students and 1,033 female students from these two schools completed the questionnaire—98 percent of the students present on the day the survey was administered. Subsequent rounds were completed by smaller numbers as a result of lower attendance and enrollment rates in the two schools; in most cases, refusal rates continued to be about 2–3 percent. At the final survey, nearly three years later, 506 male students and 695 female students answered the questionnaire.

The students used as a control group came from schools with racially mixed populations, but only the black students are used for comparison. The socioeconomic status of these students is similar to that of the students attending the two program schools. At the baseline survey, 944 male students and 1,002 female students completed the questionnaire. At the end of the project, 860 boys and 889 girls answered the questionnaire.

The baseline survey data revealed high levels of sexual activity in both the program[1] and the nonprogram schools. Almost 92 percent of boys in the ninth grade of the program junior high school were sexually active, as were 54 percent of the comparable girls. In the senior high school, 79 percent of all the girls were sexually active. Even at the lower grade levels, the percentages reporting that they were sexually experienced were relatively high: Forty-seven percent of the girls in the seventh and eighth grades had had intercourse. Approximately 71 percent of sexually active male and female students in the junior high school, and over 89 percent of those in the senior high school, said they had practiced some form of contraception. However, only 56 and 73 percent, respectively, had used any method at last intercourse. Among the sexually active girls in the seventh and eighth grades, 11 percent had been pregnant. In the ninth grade of the junior high school, this proportion rose to 20 percent, while among sexually active young women in the senior high school, 22 percent had had a pregnancy.

The pregnancy prevention program initiated in the two schools selected for the study utilized the services of a social worker and a nurse-midwife or nurse practitioner based in each of the schools. These professionals made presentations at least once a year in each homeroom. The discussions dealt with services offered in the clinic, as well as a variety of other topics related to reproductive health. For several hours each day, one or two of the staff members assigned to each school made themselves available (in the school health suite) to the students for individual or group counseling. In the afternoon, these same staff members provided services in a special clinic, which was located across the street from one of the program schools and a few blocks away from the other. In this after-school clinic, the professionals led discussion groups and offered individual and group counseling and education. Strong emphasis was placed on the development of personal responsibility, goal-setting and communication with parents. Reproductive health care—including contraceptive counseling, pregnancy testing, other medical services and referrals—was provided, as were diagnosis and referral in other health fields. Students could come simply to talk in the waiting room, to see films or to take part in group discussion, whether or not they registered for services. Young men and women could enroll in the clinic and were eligible for the services as long as they remained in school. All services were free. Thus, both educational and medical services were available to the students. A single professional staff provided continuity and a bridge for young people between the school and the clinic setting.

The pregnancy prevention program began in November 1981. The clinic opened in January 1982, and services continued to be provided until June 1984. Throughout the duration of the project, the basic sex education curriculum, which is mandated by state law and is offered in all the junior and senior high schools in Baltimore, remained in place.

Some Methodological Problems

The evaluation of school-based programs presents some special problems. First, there is likely to be a high level of movement in and out of individual schools—even those that serve specific communities—because of graduation and also because of student transfers and reassignments that take place throughout the year. Second, it is often difficult to collect data reflecting behavior "before" and "after" initiation of the program at the same time of year (when the aggregate data would, ideally, represent student samples with the same age distribution). For example, even if baseline data are collected in the fall, at the start of a new program, follow-up data may have to be gathered in the spring, in order to include the experience of students who will graduate and leave the school. Third, no two schools in any school system are truly comparable, given the wide differences that exist between them in geographic and social setting, economic, racial and gender mix, and curriculum and administrative styles and philosophies. Consequently, control schools should not be compared directly with program schools. However, they help establish the presence or absence of secular change during the experimental period.

As a result of these problems, which are common to all school-based studies, our evaluation had to address a number of issues: Because attendance at the schools varied considerably between the fall and the spring terms, a smaller sample of students was available for follow-up than at baseline. The differences could not be assumed to be completely random, since absenteeism and premature dropping out are likely to occur disproportionately among the less-motivated students. (The same potential bias would be apparent in both program and control schools.)

Second, the student sample is slightly older at the three follow-up surveys than it was at the time of the baseline survey. Generally, the age differential will have little effect on variables that are not highly age-dependent. It could have some effect on those that reflect cumulative experience; we have used life-table analysis wherever appropriate to correct for the age difference.

Third, because students move into and out of the schools, the duration of program exposure cannot be predicted by grade. For purposes of evaluation, subgroups are best defined by their actual exposure to the program. However, age distributions vary between exposure groups: Longer exposure is associated with older ages. Furthermore, exposure can vary within grade. Those who have just entered a senior high from a junior high without the pregnancy prevention program, are available for only one year of exposure. Exposure groups must, therefore, be controlled by grade level and by school (and, sometimes, by school of origin). Despite the large size of the initial sample, numbers remaining in some grade/exposure subgroups may be substantially reduced by the end of the project.

In the appendix at the end of the article (page 126), we discuss in greater detail some of the practical problems posed by the need to define appropriate groups for comparison, and explain the methodology introduced to address this need. The appendix also contains a table showing the size of the samples in the program schools at baseline and at each of the three follow-up surveys, by the student's gender and grade level.

The units of interest in this article are "exposure groups," defined as groups of students exposed to the pregnancy prevention program for zero, one, two or three years. Zero exposure is based on information obtained at the baseline survey. One-year exposure is based on data from the second round of the survey plus that subset of students interviewed in the third round who had entered the program schools in the second year of project activities. Two-year exposure includes all students in the third round of questionnaires who had attended a program school since the program's onset plus those interviewed in the fourth round who had entered the school in the program's second year. Finally, three-year exposure includes the subset of respondents in the fourth round who were exposed to the program for all three years of its operation.

Changes in Knowledge and Attitudes

Students in grades 9–12 were asked 10 questions on the correct use of specific contraceptive methods and on the risk of pregnancy. At the time of the baseline survey, female students scored an average of 6.8 correct answers; the average increased from 5.4 among those in the ninth grade to 7.4 among students in the 12th grade. Subsequent rounds of the survey show that the number of correct answers increases in all grades over the course of the program, and significantly* overall. However, the change is not dramatic, and the overall average after two or more years of exposure to the program is 7.8 correct answers. Among female students in the 11th and 12th grades, the highest level of correct knowledge reached after two or more years of exposure is 8.2. In the control schools, where correct knowledge started at levels comparable to those found in the program schools, the high point among female students does not exceed a correct average of 7.2 by the end of the program.

A significant increase in knowledge occurs among male students at all durations of exposure to the program, while the changes observed in the nonprogram schools among males and females do not achieve significance.

As a further measure of knowledge, students were asked to identify the time during the menstrual cycle when conception is most likely to occur. If the answer was "at any time during the month," this was considered as correct as "about two weeks after period begins," since either can be interpreted as a "protective" response. Table 1 (top panel) shows the trends in the percentage of female students at the program and nonprogram schools who answered the question "correctly." The table shows that among female students exposed to the program, levels of knowledge increase significantly

---

*Significance was measured by the t-test.

Table 1.

Percentage of female students correctly identifying the fertile period of the menstrual cycle; and percentages of female and male students who believe that the less-effective methods* are good for preventing pregnancy; by grade level, according to years of exposure to the program; program and nonprogram schools

Years of exposure to the program	Program schools, by grade										Nonprogram schools, by grade							
	Total†	Adjusted total†,‡	7	8	9a	9b	10a§	10b§	11	12	Total†	Adjusted total†,‡	7	8	9	10	11	12
Females correctly identifying fertile period																		
0	26.2	29.7	13.9	25.7	28.6	26.3	14.3	31.3	32.8	34.6	30.5	30.7	28.6	33.3	37.5	28.6	32.3	24.1
1	38.7	na	31.7	38.7	40.5	42.9	44.4	39.1	33.8	50.0	u	u	u	u	u	u	u	u
≥2	na	44.4	**	40.8	45.5	††	35.3	55.9	34.8	46.7	36.4	37.9	30.0	30.8	42.9	37.8	46.2	41.9
Females believing less-effective methods are good at preventing pregnancy																		
0	38.9	37.8	43.2	52.1	57.6	48.8	60.0	43.5	24.5	25.6	50.9	46.8	82.4	57.1	50.0	55.2	32.4	41.9
1	26.1	na	43.1	44.8	40.2	17.6	33.3	21.3	16.2	14.9	u	u	u	u	u	u	u	u
≥2	na	23.8	**	52.9	43.8	††	24.3	11.8	14.9	17.9	45.6	43.9	61.1	61.9	38.9	44.3	47.1	30.6
Males believing less-effective methods are good at preventing pregnancy																		
0	53.7	53.3	53.8	41.8	66.2	70.0	81.3	61.8	43.5	45.7	48.8	49.7	47.6	50.0	26.7	59.4	55.9	51.8
1	42.9	na	50.7	39.8	59.2	20.0	37.5	31.7	40.4	40.5	u	u	u	u	u	u	u	u
≥2	na	34.4	**	47.2	49.3	††	36.4	16.7	30.4	30.3	59.2	60.3	52.9	66.7	75.0	59.1	58.5	41.7

*Withdrawal, rhythm and douche.

†Standardized on the grade distribution of the program schools at the time of the baseline survey.

‡Omits grades exposed to the program for only one year.

§Grade 10a students came from the program junior high school; 10b, from junior high schools that had no program.

**These students could not have been exposed to the program for more than one year.

††Grade 9a is in the junior high. Grade 9b is the equivalent grade in the senior high school. Since no 9b students came from the program junior high school, they could not have been exposed to the program for more than one year.

Notes: In this and subsequent tables, u = unavailable; na = not applicable; and years of exposure for nonprogram students refer to the interval since the baseline survey. All differences between exposures zero and one and between zero and two or more in the program schools are statistically significant (p<0.001 or p<0.01). In the nonprogram schools, none of the changes are statistically significant. See the appendix for a further discussion of these notes.

over time,* especially among the younger girls. Among male students (not shown), knowledge of the fertile period shows a slight, though not statistically significant, upward trend. As the top panel of Table 1 also shows, among the female students attending the nonprogram schools, knowledge of the fertile period increases slightly in the course of the project period. However, the changes are not statistically significant. Among males, there is actually a decrease (not shown).

It should be noted that even in the program schools, it is rare for more than 50 percent of female students to answer correctly. There are, nevertheless, indications of a pattern of change that may be important: The acquisition of correct knowledge appears to be occurring at an earlier age, so that following exposure to the program, younger students are achieving higher scores than older students had attained prior to the intervention.

The second and third panels of Table 1 record the proportions of female and male students who consider that withdrawal, the rhythm method and douches are "good" or "very good" methods for avoiding pregnancy. A significant downward trend in the level of misperception emerges among students of both sexes, at one or more year's exposure to the program. By contrast, although there is also an insignificant decrease among girls attending the nonprogram schools, a clear trend is not evident, since some grades appear to improve their knowledge, while others regress.

The questionnaires also probed student attitudes toward three issues: the acceptability of teenage pregnancy; the "best" or ideal age to have children and to marry; and when sexual relationships are "okay." Our earlier studies of this student sample found a significant relationship between having a positive attitude toward adolescent childbearing and the ineffective practice of contraception, although only a small percentage were supportive of adolescent parenthood.[2] The present study shows little consistent change in this attitude after exposure to the program. Positive support for adolescent childbearing declines among females, but does not change in any one direction among males.

Analysis of the responses shows generally slight and inconsistent attitudinal changes in the other two areas. A large proportion (often, over 50 percent) of both male and female students cite an ideal age for childbearing that is lower than the age they consider to be ideal for marriage. After exposure to the program, the percentage declines among the girls but not among the boys. In the nonprogram schools, in contrast, there is no such change. In fact, an increase occurs among female students. On the third

---

*Measured on the basis of the Mantel-Haentszel summed chi-square. However, since the observations are not truly independent and the sample is not a probability sample, the meaning of the significance levels should be interpreted with caution. A level of $p<0.01$ is required for significance. All significance tests in Tables 1, 2 and 3 were performed on the basis of the actual numbers, by grade, not on the basis of the standardized totals.

measure—finding sexual intercourse acceptable between individuals who have just met or who date occasionally—there is no consistent change seen in the program schools, while a decline that is not statistically significant occurs among students in the nonprogram schools. These findings appear to suggest that the program occasioned less of a change in attitudes than it did in knowledge.

Changes in Behavior

In terms of behavioral change, we had predicted that in view of the very high rates of sexual activity prevailing in the study schools, it would be difficult for the program to have any impact on the timing of initiation of intercourse. The broken line in Figure 1 reflects the cumulative percentage of female students 15 years of age and older in the program senior high school who became sexually active during the course of three years of exposure to the program. The solid line reflects, for the zero-exposure group in the same school, their histories over a similar period of time, before the program was in place. It thus serves as the comparison. (The points on both curves are derived from standard life-table analysis. See the appendix for details.) The results of this comparison show an apparent postponement of first intercourse among high school students exposed to the program for three years. The median length of the delay (not shown) is seven months (from 15 years and seven months before the program to 16 years and two months afterwards). The smaller delays found after one or two years' exposure are hardly surprising, since such changes cannot be expected in a short period of time and require early precoital intervention.

Of even greater interest than the median age at first intercourse is the shape of the curves shown in Figure 1. While both curves demonstrate similarly rapid initiation of sexual intercourse between the ages of 13 and 16, at ages 14 and 15 there is a substantial difference in the proportions who have become sexually active. At age 14, for example, about two-thirds more girls had become sexually active before the program started as had done so after three years of exposure to the program.

Table 2 illustrates the effects of the program on attendance at a birth control clinic.* The table shows that the proportion of sexually active students in the program schools who attended a clinic rises at all grade levels for both male and female students. In fact, among male students in the junior high school, attendance climbs to levels that parallel those of senior high school female students prior to the program's introduction. The overall

---

*Male students were asked whether they had "ever been to a birth control clinic." Female students were asked whether they had "ever been to a clinic or doctor to get birth control."

Figure 1.
Cumulative percentage of female high school students aged 15 and older who initiated coitus during the three years before the baseline survey and during the three years before the final program survey, by age at first coitus

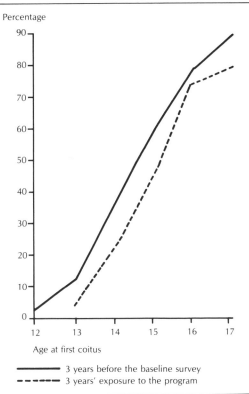

Percentage

Age at first coitus

——— 3 years before the baseline survey
- - - - - 3 years' exposure to the program

changes are statistically significant. In the control schools, no consistent changes in clinic attendance occur.

Again on the basis of life-table analysis, Figure 2 illustrates the relationship between the date of first coitus and the timing of first clinic attendance among female students exposed to the program for one year.* The graph reveals striking and highly significant differences between the "before" and "after" groups in their probability of having been to a clinic or doctor for birth control services, by month following first coitus. After one year of exposure to the program, a higher percentage of girls than before made a

*The comparison involves students involved in the program for only one year, since this is the only group not limited by age. It should be noted that the figure does not separate from the total those girls who attended the school clinic only.

Table 2.

Percentages of sexually active female and male students who had attended a birth control clinic;* by grade level, according to years of exposure to the program; and nonprogram schools

Years of exposure to the program	Program schools, by grade										Nonprogram schools, by grade							
	Total†	Adjusted total†,‡	7	8	9a	9b	10a§	10b§	11	12	Total†	Adjusted total†,‡	7	8	9	10	11	12
Females																		
0	49.4	51.9	32.7	32.8	33.3	23.8	50.0	42.5	56.9	69.3	57.6	62.7	13.3	25.0	38.5	61.2	67.6	82.8
1	63.3	na	38.2	57.3	56.1	41.0	81.8	58.7	76.0	71.6	u	u	u	u	u	u	u	u
≥2	na	70.9	**	64.5	57.1	††	62.5	70.4	75.7	75.0	55.7	59.8	16.7	20.0	47.1	55.1	71.2	75.0
Males																		
0	15.6	16.3	12.4	23.8	16.3	12.5	5.6	10.3	19.7	14.5	10.4	11.6	5.6	19.0	6.3	10.5	13.8	9.4
1	27.5	na	37.1	33.7	25.9	16.7	20.0	17.4	25.8	26.8	u	u	u	u	u	u	u	u
≥2	na	47.6	**	61.9	44.7	††	63.6	33.3	34.3	63.6	10.8	12.1	5.6	10.5	8.3	15.2	15.7	10.1

*Female students were asked whether they had "ever been to a clinic or doctor to get birth control." Males were asked whether they had "ever been to a birth control clinic."

Note: For the meaning of all other symbols, see footnotes to Table 1.

Figure 2.
Cumulative percentage of sexually active female students in grades 9–12*
who attended a birth control clinic, by month following first coitus, one
year before the baseline survey and after one year of exposure to the
program

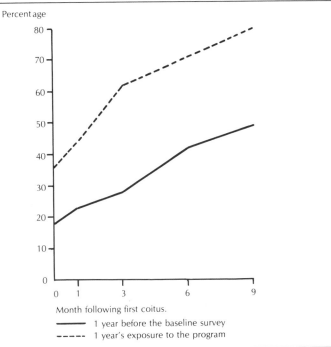

Percentage

Month following first coitus.
——— 1 year before the baseline survey
- - - - 1 year's exposure to the program

*Excludes students who initiated sexual activity more than one year before the survey.

visit while they were still virgins, and increased percentages attended a health facility in the months soon after initiation of intercourse. A similar comparison among students exposed to the program for three years (not shown) indicates that 92 percent of female students ages 15 and older had attended a professional facility by the end of the observation period. There were large increases in attendance among the younger students, and these were even greater than those found among older girls, as Table 2 indicates.

Table 3 (page 120) shows trends in the use of the pill at last intercourse among sexually active female students and in the use of any contraceptive method for which the partners are prepared in advance (i.e., any except withdrawal, rhythm or douche) among female and male students. All such methods require forethought on the part of one of the two partners and are, therefore, an indication of a certain level of preparedness for sexual intercourse.[3]

Table 3.
Percentage of sexually active female students who used the pill at last intercourse; and percentages of sexually active female and male students protected by any method requiring advance preparation* at last intercourse; by grade level, according to years of exposure to the program; program and nonprogram schools

Years of exposure to the program	Program schools, by grade										Nonprogram schools, by grade							
	Total†	Adjusted total†,‡	7	8	9a	9b	10a§	10b§	11	12	Total†	Adjusted total†,‡	7	8	9	10	11	12
Females who used the pill at last intercourse																		
0	31.5	32.9	21.6	24.6	6.5	20.0	30.0	25.2	34.1	49.1	30.7	32.7	21.4	7.7	0.0	29.8	40.3	48.4
1	37.5	na	26.0	31.5	28.1	25.6	60.0	34.6	45.6	42.4	u	u	u	u	u	u	u	u
≥2	na	49.9	**	38.6	32.2	††	50.0	47.2	50.7	61.0	34.4	35.9	20.0	25.0	31.3	22.2	37.5	52.4
Females protected by a method requiring advance preparation at last intercourse																		
0	56.9	57.3	54.9	49.2	41.3	50.0	30.0	54.1	62.0	65.6	54.7	54.9	50.0	23.1	61.5	48.9	63.9	64.1
1	67.7	na	60.3	57.3	66.7	87.2	70.0	65.4	72.8	69.7	u	u	u	u	u	u	u	u
≥2	na	76.6	**	75.4	57.6	††	79.2	75.5	72.0	87.0	54.0	53.4	60.0	60.0	56.3	37.8	43.8	71.4
Males protected by a method requiring advance preparation at last intercourse																		
0	49.0	47.9	54.1	44.6	45.8	50.0	33.3	48.9	48.7	56.3	52.2	50.6	58.8	44.4	62.5	43.2	45.8	60.6
1	59.5	na	59.1	53.6	61.0	33.3	71.4	55.4	61.0	68.3	u	u	u	u	u	u	u	u
≥2	na	55.6	**	64.9	43.4	††	78.9	41.7	62.1	65.5	49.7	51.9	38.9	42.1	54.5	54.7	55.3	50.8

*Any method except withdrawal, rhythm or douche.
Note: For the meaning of all other symbols, see footnotes to Table 1.

At the baseline survey, we found that pill use generally increases with age, as might have been expected. However, after exposure to the program, the percentage using increases further still among all grade levels. Differences in both time periods are statistically significant. Moreover, even with brief exposure to the program, the increases are more pronounced among younger than among older students. With increased exposure to the program, the differentials by age diminish. Finally, the table shows, among younger students, pill use at last coitus increases with program exposure to levels higher than those reported by some groups of older students before the program began. This accelerated adoption of effective contraception can be expected in the long run to reduce the high risks of pregnancy experienced by young women who initiate sexual activity in their early, postpubertal years.

As Table 3 also indicates, the difference between younger and older students that was noted in use of the pill is smaller for use of all methods requiring advance preparation. This finding is a result of the widespread use of the condom at younger ages. Increases in the use of these protective methods are significant for both males and females. In the nonprogram schools, by comparison, use of these methods declines in seven of the grade/sex groups and increases in five.

Use of no contraceptive method at last intercourse is reduced to extremely low levels after exposure to the program (not shown). In all instances except one subgroup of one grade, fewer than 20 percent of female students exposed to the risk of pregnancy were unprotected by any method at the time of their most recent coitus, after exposure to the program for two or more years. This is true even at the seventh and eighth grade levels, at ages often associated with poor contraceptive use. In contrast, in three of the grades at the nonprogram schools, 44–49 percent of the students were using no method of birth control at all, and only one grade reached the level of protection found in the program schools.

Pregnancy Rates

What effect, if any, do these significant changes in clinic attendance and contraceptive practice have on pregnancy rates? Among the issues involved in calculating changes in schoolwide pregnancy rates from aggregate data is the fact that the Baltimore public school system allows students who become pregnant to transfer to a special school for pregnant girls. Since lists of these transfers from the program and control schools were available, this issue could be addressed: We were able to ascertain which of these young women had, in fact, been part of one of the exposure cohorts, even though they were no longer attending the study schools when follow-up rounds of the survey were administered. These girls, unsurprisingly, represent from 10 percent to 20 percent of all pregnant students reported in each school year and an even higher proportion of those who carried to term. By adding the girls who went to the special school to their original cohorts, when and where appropriate, and by determining their correct exposure group, using life-table analysis, we can more precisely estimate the effects of the program on pregnancies. (In this part of the analysis, the second round of the surveys constitutes the baseline, in order to ensure strictly comparable age distributions. Most of the pregnant girls in round 2 had, in fact, conceived before the clinic opened. On the other hand, it is possible that by using round 2, we may minimize program impact, since the pregnancy rates *could* have begun to fall in the very first months of the project.)

Figure 3 is based on a series of life-table analyses and shows the cu-

Figure 3.
Cumulative percentage of sexually active females in grades 9–12 of the program and nonprogram schools who became pregnant during 16, 20 or 28 months prior to the baseline survey or subsequent survey, by duration of program exposure; and percentage changes in these proportions

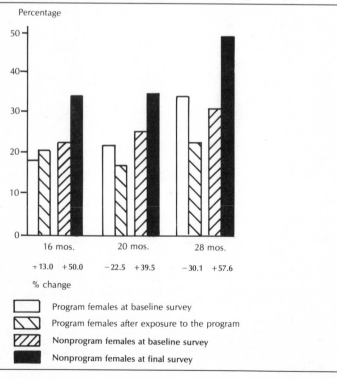

mulative percentages of sexually active students in grades 9–12 of the program and nonprogram schools who became pregnant during the 16-, 20- or 28-month period prior to the survey of interest. For the program schools, the 16-month data are based on information obtained in round 3. The findings for 20 and 28 months are based on round 4. For the nonprogram schools, the comparison is between the data from the baseline and final surveys. (For further details, see the appendix.) As the figure reveals, among students exposed to the program, there appears to have been an increase in pregnancies of 13.0 pecent after 16 months of exposure to the program. Among nonprogram students, the equivalent increase is 50.0 percent. However, after 20 months, the conception rate falls by 22.5 percent among program students, whereas it rises by 39.5 percent among nonprogram girls. Finally, after 28 months, the pregnancy rate declines by 30.1 percent, whereas it increases by 57.6 percent in the schools that had no pregnancy prevention program. Pregnancy data were subjected to many types of analysis, including examinations of pregnancies in consecutive 12-month periods and comparison of differentials by outcome of pregnancy. All confirmed the conclusion that the program led to decreases in the pregnancy rates of these 9-th–12th-grade students.

Because the numbers of sexually active students in the seventh and eighth grades were small, and because we have much more limited information on their pregnancies, it is difficult to evaluate changes among these students. There appear, however, to be small reductions in pregnancy rates among girls 15 years old and younger.

Concurrently, however, larger increases in pregnancy rates appear to have taken place in the nonprogram schools. We believe, therefore, that the program assisted these younger teenagers in avoiding the kinds of increases observed citywide, and even lead to some decrease in their pregnancies.

Conclusions

The brief, though intensive, pregnancy prevention program introduced in two Baltimore schools has demonstrated significant changes in several areas of adolescent knowledge and behavior—changes that have major implications for the formulation of public policy and for program design. The results reported in this article are based on the school populations as a whole, and do not compare the individuals who used the program services with those who did not. It is highly noteworthy, therefore, that the differentials are nonetheless statistically significant, and reflect a broad impact on the school community.

Over the course of the two and a half years that the program existed, changes in sexual and contraceptive knowledge occurred. These are both areas in which it has already been demonstrated that educational programs can make a difference.[4] The rapid effect on clinic use exerted by an intervention program designed to supplement the basic sex education program already in place suggests that it was the accessibility of the staff and of the clinic, rather than any "new" information about contraception, that encouraged the students to obtain services.

Our study has shown attitudes to be somewhat more resistant to change than practice, but in this area there was less room for change to occur. As we reported earlier, support for adolescent childbearing or for casual sex was already very low in this school population before the program began.[5] This seemed to suggest that more overall improvement was to be gained by helping students holding positive attitudes toward pregnancy prevention translate those attitudes into action than by attempting to change the attitudes of the few who do not share that view. With majority opinion already supportive of contraception and delayed childbearing, that is apparently what the program accomplished.

While the changes in the age at first intercourse are not large, they are substantial enough—in the direction of delay—to refute charges that access to such services as those provided by the program encourages early sexual activity. The program's ability to effect any further changes may well have been limited by the brevity of the project and by the age of the students when they were first reached. The fact that age at first intercourse was delayed at all is impressive, and particularly important in view of the demonstrated high risks of early exposure to pregnancy.[6]

Similarly, the results indicating that students attended clinics sooner after initiating sexual activity than had been the case are important. The project appears to demonstrate that if students in junior high schools are given access to nearby services and if they are offered information and continuity of care, they will use such services, and at levels comparable to those shown by older teenagers. That was clearly the case in this demonstration project, where confidential services were provided free of cost and in a sympathetic setting. Furthermore, the percentage of students going to a clinic or doctor before their first intercourse increased, as did attendance during the first months of sexual activity. Both these measures of preventive behavior were low at the time of the baseline survey, as they were among clinic patients observed in an earlier study,[7] and both increased markedly.

One of the most striking findings from the project is the demonstration that boys in the junior high school used the clinic as freely as girls of the same age. In view of the growing call for research into ways of attracting male clients to such facilities, the interest shown by these boys appears to be of some importance.

The changes in contraceptive use demonstrated by the evaluation are promising. Again, the results among the younger students suggest that early risk of pregnancy can be reduced with early attendance at a clinic. Use of the condom did not change consistently, but appeared to fluctuate with the use of female methods in such a way that the overall use of all methods requiring advance preparation increased significantly.

Increased and prompt clinic attendance and the resulting increased use of effective methods of contraception appear to have had a significant impact on pregnancy levels. The full extent of this impact may not have been fully realized by the time follow-up was completed. Each of the measures we used confirms the finding of a reduction in pregnancy rates among older teenagers and a halt in the rapid increases—by some measures, a decrease—in the rates among younger adolescents. In the face of rising rates in many U.S. cities, the marked reduction in pregnancy demonstrated here is to be welcomed.

As successful as this program appears to have been, a longer period than that involved here is probably needed to achieve and to measure the full impact of interventions such as these. Many effects may not be quick in coming, and although our study reports many significant effects, one would hope that with time, even more young people might be affected. Perhaps the evidence we present will encourage the investment of funds and energies in similar programs, over a longer term.

Furthermore, early program exposure is clearly of some importance; interventions will have to take place before young people develop behavior that places them at risk of early, postpubertal conception. The effects of this program apparently were somewhat greater among younger than among older students. One of its major effects, indeed, is that it appears to have encouraged the younger sexually active teenagers to develop levels of knowledge and patterns of behavior usually associated only with older adolescents. This accelerated protective behavior, coupled with evidence that first coitus was not encouraged but, in fact, postponed, should provide solid support to the current movement toward the introduction of school-based clinics. The model described here is a combined school and clinic operation that offers full reproductive health services and that is located close to, but not in, the school. When two schools are close enough to share a clinic, this may be a particularly economical model; further analysis of the component services may suggest an even more parsimonious design that could achieve many of the same results.

In conclusion, these findings suggest the efficacy of a program with pregnancy prevention as an explicit objective. Such a model requires a program and a staff capable of addressing a wide range of reproductive health issues. It does not preclude a broader range of adolescent health services (since these, too, are often badly needed), but it does suggest that meeting the sexual concerns, medical needs and contraceptive requirements of high school boys and girls is in itself an extremely challenging and demanding responsibility for program designers. More broad-based initiatives would, no doubt, have to include in their staffs some health educators, social workers, nurses or doctors with a strong commitment to the reproductive health of young people if they seek to replicate these results.

Why did this program work? Access to high-quality, free services was probably crucial to its success. Professional counseling, education and open communication were, no doubt, also important. All these factors appear to have created an atmosphere that allowed teenagers to translate their attitudes into constructive preventive behavior. Precisely which separate components of the program contributed most to its success remains to be determined. Our understanding of similar school-based services for young people may well depend on the willingness of providers to scrutinize their interventions closely, on the ability of researchers to evaluate those interventions and on the cooperation of schools in making available the types of data needed to carry out such evaluations.

Appendix

●*The tables.* Problems associated with movement into and out of schools are common to all school-based studies; each setting will involve some local differences, although the specific details may vary. In this case, because students graduated from the junior and the senior high schools involved in the project, because a new middle school was opened in the vicinity of the two schools during the course of the project, and because of the normal flow of new students into all grades, the sample population had a constantly fluctuating composition. In order to allow for these aspects of the study population, the data are controlled by the student's grade level (as a proxy for age) and by exposure to the program.

This treatment also allows us to deal with a specific problem affecting only one exposure of one grade: At the time of the final round of the survey in the program schools, the 12th-grade sample was biased, because a few sections omitted on that day turned out to be nonrandomly selected. These sections included the most motivated, advanced students, thereby making comparisons with rounds 1, 2 and 3 of the survey invalid. To correct for this problem, for the 12th-grade group in the category "two or more years," those exposed for three years are excluded from the analysis.

Thus, it can be seen that both artifacts of the research design and particulars of the schools must be considered in establishing appropriate groups for comparison. Analysis should be restricted only to those subgroups which can legitimately be compared.

Appendix Table 1 (page 127) shows the number of students in each sample cell, by gender, grade level and length of exposure to the program.

Appendix Table 1.
Number of program-school students surveyed, by years of exposure to the program and gender, and average age of students, according to grade level

Measure	Total	Grade Level							
		7	*8*	*9a**	*9b†*	*10a‡*	*10b§*	*11*	*12*
YEARS OF EXPOSURE									
0									
Male	667	148	118	109	11	20	98	85	78
Female	1,033	125	151	103	44	17	209	175	209
1									
Male	697	194	112	93	17	16	151	68	46
Female	1,146	195	152	103	78	16	319	156	127
2									
Male	352	na	115	59	na	15	13	109	41
Female	601	na	103	62	na	17	79	241	99
3									
Male	61	na	na	39	na	9	na	13	na
Female	96	na	na	31	na	22	na	43	na
AVERAGE AGE (IN YEARS)									
Male	15.4	13.8	14.7	15.6	15.1	15.8	16.0	17.0	17.8
Female	15.7	13.6	14.4	15.3	14.9	15.8	15.8	16.8	17.8

*Junior high school students only.

†Senior high school students only.

‡Students who came to the program senior high school from the program junior high school.

§Students who came to the program senior high school from other junior high schools.

In the control schools, the distributions remained virtually unchanged between the baseline and final survey.

In the appendix table, and in the earlier tables, grades 9a and 9b are the ninth grades of the junior high school and senior high school, respectively. Grades 10a and 10b are the 10th graders who came from the program junior high school and from all other junior high schools, respectively. In the calculation of the totals, distributions are standardized on the grade distribution of the program schools at the time of the baseline survey. The adjusted totals, similarly standardized, omit the grades exposed for only one year (grades 7 and 9b in the program schools, and grade 7 in the nonprogram school), and are used for comparisons between zero and two or more years' exposure. Mantel-Haentszel summed chi-square tests are used to calculate p values, on the basis of actual numbers by grade. We have imposed a strict significance level of p<0.01.

• *Figures 1 and 2.* In calculating age at first intercourse and the lag between first intercourse and clinic attendance, we used regular life-table analysis.

For the program group, the analysis is restricted to the subset of female students in the program schools who were not sexually active prior to the program. This information is based upon the student's responses to detailed questions on sexual activity and the timing of first intercourse. Age restrictions are also imposed in order to ensure comparability between samples. The comparison group, therefore, involves the experience of students of similar age, followed for a period of comparable time, who attended the program schools before the project was introduced.

• *Figure 3*. In the calculation of pregnancy rates, it seemed important to include those students who transferred to the special school for pregnant teenagers after conceiving. Because we had no information on their exact month of first intercourse, we had to make certain assumptions in order to utilize life-tables to calculate pregnancy rates. We assumed that these students had initiated sexual activity 13 months before they become pregnant, because 13 months is the average delay between first coitus and conception observed among all the pregnant students, in both the program and the nonprogram schools, for whom we had complete documentation in the baseline data. We were able to establish the month of conception among these young women by means of information on the estimated date of confinement provided by the staff of the school for pregnant teenagers.*

With this imputed information about the month of first intercourse (which we also used for the girls in the aggregate data who had a pregnancy but did not report a date of first coitus), we were able to include these girls in our calculations of pregnancy rates, which were thus made for all sexually active students in the program and the nonprogram schools, using increment-decrement life-table analysis. The estimates were controlled for length of exposure to the program, and equivalent durations (16 months, 20 months and 28 months) among students attending the program and nonprogram schools, respectively. Thus, the pregnancy experiences of young women in all of the schools were reconstructed for periods of 16, 20 and 28 months prior to the survey. The resulting life-table probabilities apply, then, to subgroups whose lengths of exposure to the program may represent quite different circumstances. For example, an exposure of 16 months' duration means that the student attended school during the initial start-up period (January 1982—June 1982), had a summer break, and completed another academic year (ending with the survey in the spring). All information on these young women comes from the third round of the survey. The 20-month exposure group attended the program schools for two full academic years, separated by a summer. The 28-month group went through the initial start-up period, two full academic years and two summers. Both sets of infor-

*The authors are grateful to Rosetta Stith, principal of the Pacquin School for pregnant girls, and to Loretta Bryant, assistant principal, for their assistance.

mation for these two last groups come from the final round of the survey, carried out in the spring of 1984. Some of the pregnancies reported among the 16-month exposure group also appear among the 28-month group (taken from the third and fourth rounds of the survey, respectively), but the 20-month group remains independent of both of the other exposure groups.

With regard to the problem of school dropouts, there is no reason to believe that the proportion of dropouts who left school *because* of a pregnancy changed over time. If the total number of dropouts did not change during the program—and, specifically, the numbers in the schools' categories of dropouts in which pregnancy-related drop-outs are likely to appear—then the percentage pregnant among them should not change enough to affect our calculations. In fact, there was little variation in the numbers in these categories dropping out before, during or after the program: Numbers remained between eight and 10 in the junior high school, and between 21 and 23 in the senior high school in each of the three program years. Therefore, we feel justified in omitting these young women from our calculations.

References

1. L. S. Zabin, M. B. Hirsch, E. A. Smith, R. Streett and J. B. Hardy, "Adolescent Pregnancy Prevention Program: A Model for Research and Evaluation," *Journal of Adolescent Health Care*, 7:77, 1986.
2. L. S. Zabin, E. A. Smith and M. B. Hirsch, "Correlates of Effective Contraception Among Black Inner-City High School Students," final report, National Institute of Child Health and Human Development, May 1985.
3. Ibid.
4. D. Kirby, J. Alter and P. Scales, *Analysis of U.S. Sex Education and Evaluation Methods*, U.S. Department of Health, Education, and Welfare, Washington, D.C., 1979; and D. Kirby, "Evaluating Sexuality Education," *Independent School*, 41:21, 1981
5. L. S. Zabin, M. B. Hirsch, E. A. Smith and J. B. Hardy, "Adolescent Sexual Attitudes and Behaviors: Are They Consistent?" *Family Planning Perspectives*, 16:181, 1984.
6. L. S. Zabin, J. F. Kantner and M. Zelnik, "The Risk of Adolescent Pregnancy in the First Months of Intercourse," *Family Planning Perspectives*, 11:215, 1979.
7. L. S. Zabin and S. D. Clark, "Why They Wait: A Study of Teenage Family Planning Clinic Patients," *Family Planning Perspectives*, 13:205, 1981.

Appendix B
Parental Notification Form

Memo: To Parents of ——————— 8th and 9th Grade Students

From: ——————— Pregnancy Prevention Program and ——————— Principal

One out of every three babies born in ——————— is born to a teenager. As parents, we know what that means to our children. We know that most teenage parents:

1. Never finish school
2. Have lower paying jobs throughout life
3. Have taken on more responsibility than they can handle at such a young age.

The whole family pays the price.

Some of our young people are at risk, many are not. But what *every* student thinks and feels and knows is important to us, if we are to help them and understand them while they are still young.

We invite you to join us in a new special project to reduce the number of teenage pregnancies. We are placing some extra staff in ——————— to work with the school and parents to try to meet the problem. You will be hearing more from us soon and we hope you'll get involved.

In order to plan our program, we must find out a great deal about *all* our young students. We must find out how many students are in danger of becoming pregnant, how much they know about how to prevent pregnancy, and how they feel about teenage pregnancy. To do this we are giving all students in the 8th and 9th grade of ——————— an anonymous, very personal questionnaire on September 28th and 29th. No names or other identifying information will be allowed. Nobody in the school or at ———— ———— will ever know how any one student answered.

The cooperation of every student in these grades will help us find ways to serve young people all over the United States. We hope everybody will take part. If you have any questions or if you do not want your child to participate, please call us at ———————— anytime between 9 a.m. and 6 p.m. on Thursday, September 24th, or Friday, September 25th.

As a member of the ———————— family we deeply appreciate your continued support of this important program. Together we can make a difference in helping our children make a life for themselves before they make another life.

Appendix C
The Survey Instruments

<u>FEMALE VERSION (A)</u>

1	4	3			

*Questions that are omitted or very different from the male version are marked with an asterisk.

HEALTH QUESTIONNAIRE

ALL ANSWERS ARE CONFIDENTIAL

Please *DO NOT* write your name on this form. This questionnaire is being given to young people in high school in order
to find out ways to serve their needs better. We hope you will
help other young people and yourselves by giving us honest
answers to these very personal questions. It is entirely voluntary and confidential, and no one in school will see it. We
thank you for your cooperation.

START HERE

    A. How many older brothers (real or step) do you have? _____

    B. How many younger brothers (real or step) do you have? _____

    C. How many older sisters (real or step) do you have? _____

    D. How many younger sisters (real or step) do you have? _____

    1. How old are you? _____

    2. When were you born? _____ ____ ____
                            MONTH DAY YEAR

    3. What grade are you in? _____

    4. How many years have you gone to *this* school? (CHECK ONE)

       Since the _____ 7th grade, _____ 8th grade, _____ 9th grade,

                 _____ 10th grade, _____ 11th grade, or _____ 12th grade

    5. What school did you go to before you came here? _____

6. What was your grade average in school this year? (CHECK *ONE*)

_____ A

_____ B

_____ C

_____ D

_____ Below D

7. Are you . . .

_____ Black?

_____ White?

_____ Oriental?

_____ American Indian?

_____ Other? _____

8. Are you Hispanic? _____ Yes _____ No

9. Are you . . .

_____ Single?

_____ Married?

_____ Divorced or Separated?

10. What is your religion? (CHECK *ONE*)

_____ Jehovah's Witness _____ Greek Orthodox

_____ Holiness _____ Muslim

_____ Catholic _____ None

_____ Jewish _____ Protestant: Which group? _____

_____ Other: Which? _____

11. How many times have you been to a religious service in the last 4 weeks?

_____

12. Have you ever been in foster care?

_____ Yes How many _____ weeks OR _____ months OR

_____ No _____ years? (FILL IN *ONLY ONE*),

13. Do you expect to go on for more education after you finish school?

_____ Yes _____ No

IF YES: Do you expect to:

_____ Graduate from a two-year college

_____ Graduate from a four-year college

_____ Finish college and go on to some kind of graduate school

_____ Get some kind of job training

Do you expect to enter Military Service? _____ Yes _____ No

14. Did you have a job last summer for pay in which you worked at least 20 hours a week?

 _____ Yes _____ No What was the job you had? _____

 _____

15. Are you going with a boy? _____ Yes _____ No
 IF YES: How long have you been going with him?

 How many _____ weeks OR _____ months OR _____ years? (FILL IN *ONLY ONE*)

 How old is he? _____ years old

16. Do you plan to get married to someone you are dating now?

 _____ Yes _____ No

17. What do you think is the best age for a woman to get married?

 _____ years old

 What do you think is the best age for a man to get married?

 _____ years old

attitudes

18. Having sex (going all the way) is okay if the boy and girl (CHECK AS MANY AS YOU WANT)

 _____ Are married

 _____ Plan to marry soon

 _____ Are going steady

 _____ Are dating often

 _____ Are dating occasionally

 _____ Just met

19. Whose job is it to see that a girl doesn't get pregnant when having sex?

 _____ The girl's

 _____ The boy's

 _____ Both

 _____ Neither

20. Having a baby when you are in high school

 _____ Is not a problem at all.

 _____ Is not a problem because your family helps.

 _____ Is a problem but it's okay.

 _____ Is a problem for you and the baby but *not* the father of the baby.

 _____ Is a problem for you, the baby *and* for the father of the baby.

21. What is the best age for a girl or boy to have sex for the first time?

 Best age for a girl _____ years old

 Best age for a boy _____ years old

22. Where is the *one* place you learned *most* about sex and birth control? (CHECK *ONLY ONE*)

_____ Parent

_____ Girlfriend

_____ Boyfriend

_____ Other family members

_____ Clinic

_____ Books, etc.

_____ School

_____ Other: _____

23. How good do you think each of these ways are at *keeping a girl from getting pregnant?* (FOR *EACH* WAY, PUT A CHECK MARK IN *ONE* OF THE COLUMNS.)

	NEVER HEARD OF IT	VERY GOOD	GOOD	FAIR	POOR
Diaphragm					
Condom (rubber)					
IUD (loop, coil)					
Rhythm (safe time of month)					
Foam, Cream, Jelly, Suppository					
Pill					
Withdrawal (pulling out)					
Douche					

24. How many of your friends (girls) have had sex?

_____ None of my friends

_____ Few of my friends

_____ Most of my friends

_____ All of my friends

25. Have you ever had V.D.?   _____ Yes _____ No

IF YES: CHECK which one: Herpes _____

Gonorrhea _____

Other: What was it? _____

When was the last time you had V.D.? _____ ____
MONTH YEAR

26. What do you think is the best age for a woman to have her first baby?

_____ yrs. old

What do you think is the best age for a man to become a father?

_____ yrs. old

27. (CHECK EACH SENTENCE TRUE OR FALSE, OR DON'T KNOW)

	TRUE	FALSE	DON'T KNOW
A. The birth control pill is safe if it is prescribed by a doctor after a check-up.	_____	_____	_____
B. Condoms (rubbers) can be used without foam or jelly.	_____	_____	_____
C. Using a condom can help prevent V.D.	_____	_____	_____
D. Withdrawal or "pulling out" can help prevent V.D.	_____	_____	_____
E. "Pulling out" prevents pregnancy only if the man pulls out before he comes.	_____	_____	_____
F. An abortion can be done safely and easily by a doctor during the first 12 weeks of pregnancy.	_____	_____	_____
G. A 12-year-old girl can get pregnant right after she has her first menstrual period.	_____	_____	_____
H. Douche (washing out the vagina) is a method of birth control.	_____	_____	_____
I. The rhythm method only works if you *know* the safe time of the month and have sex only then.	_____	_____	_____
J. A woman can get pregnant even if she has sex only once.	_____	_____	_____

*28. Have you ever been to a clinic or doctor to get birth control?

_____ Yes _____ No

IF YES: When was the *first* time you got birth control from a clinic or doctor?

_____
MONTH YEAR

If you can't remember the month, was it:

_____ Winter (January/February/March)

_____ Spring (April/May/June)

_____ Summer (July/August/September)

in _____
YEAR

How old were you? _____ years old

Was it a _____ hospital or hospital clinic.

_____ Self Center

_____ other clinic

_____ private doctor, or

_____ somewhere else? Where? _____

*29. On that first visit, did you

_____ go for birth control

_____ go for something else, but they gave you birth control, too.

What method of birth control did you receive? _____

How long did you use that method? _____

Why did you stop? _____

Are you using birth control pills now? _____ Yes _____ No

*30. Have you ~~come on yet~~ (had your first monthly period)? *yet*
_____ Yes _____ No

IF YES: When was your first monthly period? _____ _____
                                              MONTH YEAR

How old were you? _____

If you do not remember the month, was it:

_____ Winter (January/February/March)

_____ Spring (April/May/June)   in ____

_____ Summer (July/August/September)   YEAR

_____ Fall (October/November/December)

31. How old is your mother? _____ years old

How old is your mother's *oldest* child? _____ years old

32. Have any of your friends been pregnant? _____ Yes _____ No
_____ Don't know

Have any of them thought they were pregnant when they weren't?

_____ Yes _____ No _____ Don't know

33. Have any of your friends had a baby? _____ Yes _____ No
_____ Don't know

34. Have any of your friends had an abortion? _____ Yes _____ No
_____ Don't know

*35. Please check any reason that has ever made it hard for you to get a birth control method from a clinic: (CHECK AS MANY AS YOU WANT).

_____ (A) It's never been hard. GO TO QUESTION #36

_____ (B) I was afraid my family would find out if I went.

_____ (C) I wanted to get pregnant.

_____ (D) My boyfriend didn't want me to use birth control.

_____ (E) I was waiting until I had a closer relationship with my boyfriend.

_____ (F) I thought it was wrong to use birth control.

_____ (G) I thought it was dangerous to use birth control.

_____ (H) I thought I was too young to get pregnant.

_____ (I) I didn't think I had sex often enough to get pregnant.

_____ (J) I thought you weren't allowed to get birth control until you were older.

_____ (K) I was afraid to be examined.

_____ (L) I thought it cost too much.

_____ (M) I didn't know where to get birth control.

_____ (N) Because I had sex with someone in my family (or close to my family) and I didn't want to talk about it.

_____ (O) Because I was forced to have sex; I didn't want to do it.

_____ (P) Because I didn't expect to have sex; it was always a surprise.

_____ (Q) I thought the kind of birth control I was using was good enough to keep me from getting pregnant.

_____ (R) I didn't need to because I wasn't having sex.

_____ (S) I never wanted any kind of birth control.

NOW, WRITE THE LETTER THAT IS NEXT TO YOUR *MOST IMPORTANT REASON* IN THIS BOX

36. Have you ever had sex (intercourse, gone all the way) with a boy?

_____ Yes _____ No

How old were you the first time? _____ years old
IF YOU *HAVE EVER HAD SEX WITH A BOY*, GO ON TO THE NEXT QUESTION.
IF YOU *HAVE NEVER HAD SEX WITH A BOY*, GO ON TO QUESTION #53.

How old was he? _____ years old

When was the first time you had sex with a boy? _____ _____
MONTH YEAR

If you do not remember the month, was it:

_____ Winter (January/February/March)

_____ Spring (April/May/June)

_____ Summer (July/August/September)

_____ Fall (October/November/December)

in _____
YEAR

37. Did you or your partner *ever* do anything to keep you from getting pregnant when you had sex? _____ Yes _____ No

IF YES: Did you do anything to keep yourself from getting pregnant the *first* time you had sex? _____ Yes _____ No

Since you first did anything to keep from getting pregnant, have you done something: _____ Always

_____ Most of the time

_____ Not very much

_____ Never

38. Check any method *you* have ever used while having sex: (CHECK AS MANY AS YOU HAVE USED, EVEN IF YOU ONLY USED IT ONCE OR TWICE).

_____ Pill

_____ IUD (loop, coil)

_____ Cream, jelly, foam or suppository

_____ Diaphragm

_____ Rhythm (safe time of month)

_____ Douche

_____ Other: Please describe it: _____

Check any method of birth control *your partner* has ever used while having sex with you:

_____ Condom (rubber)

_____ Withdrawal (pulling out)

_____ Other: Please describe it: _____

39. When was the last time you had sex?

_____ _____ when I was _____ years old.
MONTH YEAR

How old was your partner? _____ years old

At that time were you: _____ engaged to him

_____ going with him

_____ just friends with him

_____ just met him

_____ other: _____

40. What method (or methods) of birth control did you *or your partner* use the *last* time you had sex?

_____ None, no method was used by me or my partner

_____ Pill

_____ IUD (loop, coil)

_____ Cream, jelly, foam or suppository

_____ Diaphragm

_____ Rhythm (safe time of month)

_____ Douche

_____ Condom (rubber)

_____ Withdrawal (pulling out)

_____ Other: Please describe it: _____

41. In the *last four weeks*, how many times did you have sex? _____

What is the *most* times you ever had sex in one month? _____

With how many boys have you ever had sex? _____

42. Have you ever thought you were pregnant when you really weren't?

_____ Yes _____ No

How many times has that happened? _____
(NUMBER)

*43. Have you ever had a baby? _____ Yes _____ No

Have you ever had an abortion? _____ Yes _____ No

Have you ever had a miscarriage? _____ Yes _____ No

Are you pregnant now? _____ Yes _____ No

IF YOU HAVE *NEVER* BEEN PREGNANT AT ALL, GO TO QUESTION #52, ON THE NEXT PAGE.
IF YOU HAVE *EVER* BEEN PREGNANT, GO RIGHT ON TO QUESTION #44.

*44. How many babies have you had? _____

How many abortions have you had? _____

How many miscarriages have you had? _____

*45. The *first* time you were pregnant, what did you do?

I had a baby in (MONTH) _____, 19____.

I had an abortion in (MONTH) _____, 19____.

I had a miscarriage in (MONTH) _____, 19____.

I am _____ months pregnant now.
(NUMBER)

*46. The *last* time you were pregnant, what did you do?

I had a baby in (MONTH) _____, 19____.

I had an abortion in (MONTH) _____, 19____.

I had a miscarriage in (MONTH) _____, 19____.

I am _____ months pregnant now.
     (NUMBER)

*47. In the last year (12 months) How many babies have you had?   _____

How many abortions have you had?   _____

How many miscarriages have you had?   ____

*48. Have you ever become pregnant on purpose; not by accident?

_____ Yes _____ No

When was the last time this happened?   _____ ____
                                         MONTH YEAR

49. When you got pregnant last time (or this time), what method or methods of birth control were you *or your boyfriend* using at the time you got pregnant?

_____ None, no method was used by me or my partner

_____ Pill

_____ IUD (loop, coil)

_____ Cream, jelly, foam or suppository

_____ Diaphragm

_____ Rhythm (safe time of month)

_____ Douche

_____ Condom (rubber)

_____ Withdrawal (pulling out)

_____ Other: Please describe it: _____

50. Before you got pregnant the last time (or this time), did *you* want to get pregnant? _____ Yes _____ No

Did *your boyfriend* want you to get pregnant? _____ Yes _____ No

51. If you are pregnant now, what are your plans?

_____ Put the baby up for adoption.

_____ Have someone else in our family raise it.

_____ Have an abortion (stop the pregnancy)

_____ Have the baby and raise it myself.

_____ Have the baby and raise it together, but we don't plan to marry.

_____ Have the baby, get married (are married) and raise it together.

_____ Other: _____

52. Think about the time *before* you ever had sex.

    Did you think having sex could make a girl pregnant?

    _____ Yes _____ No

    Did you think you would have a good chance of getting pregnant if you had sex? _____ Yes _____ No

    Did you ever think of getting birth control for yourself?

    _____ Yes _____ No

    Did you or your boyfriend ever talk about the chance of your getting pregnant? _____ Yes _____ No

    Did you or your boyfriend ever talk about any kind of birth control?

    _____ Yes _____ No

53. What do you think *now?*

    Do you think having sex can make a girl pregnant?

    _____ Yes _____ No

    Do you think you would have a good chance of getting pregnant if you had sex? _____ Yes _____ No

    Have you thought of getting birth control for yourself?

    _____ Yes _____ No

    Did you and your boyfriend ever talk about the chance of your getting pregnant? _____ Yes _____ No

    Did you and your boyfriend ever talk about any kind of birth control?

    _____ Yes _____ No

54. Do you think that *you* could get pregnant easily if you have sex?

    _____ Yes _____ No _____ Don't Know

    IF NO: Why not? _____

    _____

55. If you got pregnant by a boy *you don't love*, would you:

    _____ Have an abortion (stop the pregnancy).

    _____ Have the baby and put it up for adoption.

    _____ Have the baby and raise it yourself.

    _____ Have the baby, not get married and raise it together.

    _____ Have the baby, get married and raise it together.

    _____ Other: _____

56. If I got pregnant, I think my mother

    _____ Would really be glad it happened.

    _____ Would not be glad, but wouldn't mind.

    _____ Would be upset, but not for long.

    _____ Would be very upset.

57. Would your parents like it or not like it if you (CIRCLE YOUR ANSWERS.)

    Did not graduate from high school? LIKE NOT LIKE WOULDN'T CARE

    Had sex with your boyfriend?   LIKE NOT LIKE WOULDN'T CARE

    Became pregnant (while in school)? LIKE NOT LIKE WOULDN'T CARE

    If you got pregnant while you were in school, would your parents want

    you to have: _____ a baby or _____ an abortion?

58. Getting pregnant is a good way to show people you are an adult.

    _____ True _____ False

59. In general, children born to teenage parents have more problems than

    children born to parents in their 20's. _____ True _____ False

60. It's important to be married before you have a baby.

    _____ True _____ False

61. How many children do you want to have? _____
    (NUMBER)

62. Do you smoke cigarettes?

    _____ Never

    _____ Yes, occasionally; less than 1 a day

    _____ 1 to 9 a day

    _____ 1/2 pack a day; but less than 20

    _____ A pack or more a day

63. When did you first begin to smoke cigarettes?

    _____ _____ when I was _____ years old.
    MONTH YEAR

64. Do you want to get married some day? _____ Yes _____ No

65. Suppose you got pregnant in the next six months, how would you feel?
    I would feel:

    _____ *Very* upset

    _____ A little upset

    _____ Not upset

    _____ Happy

    _____ *Very* happy

66. Having a baby now would be a problem to me because (CHECK AS MANY AS YOU WANT).

——— It would cost too much.

——— I'd have a hard time finishing school.

——— I'd have a hard time going to college.

——— It would make it hard to get married.

——— It would make it hard to get a job.

——— I don't want anyone to know I'm having sex

——— No problem

——— Other: _____

67. I think it is all right to have an abortion (CHECK AS MANY AS YOU WANT).

——— If the woman has been raped.

——— If the woman is very young; under 15.

——— If the pregnancy is a risk to the woman's health.

——— It the unborn child is known to be deformed.

——— If the woman doesn't want a baby for any reason of her own.

——— Never

	Yes	No	How many times last month?	(PUT NUMBER)
68. Do you drink beer or wine?				
Do you drink hard liquor?				
Do you smoke pot (reefers)?				
Do you use any other street drugs?				

substance abuse

69. Have you taken this Questionnaire before? ——— Yes ——— No

   IF YES: How many times before this one? ——— one time

   ——— two times ——— three times

70. Does any adult in your home work regularly for pay?

——— Yes ——— No

Is your family on Medical Assistance now? ——— Yes ——— No
Does anyone in your household get a Social Service check now?

——— Yes ——— No

economic situation

Does your family get food stamps now? ——— Yes ——— No
Does anyone in your household get an unemployment check now?

——— Yes ——— No

to pg. 152

71. Did you know there were people from the Self Center you could talk to privately *in School?* _____ Yes _____ No

72. Have the people from the Self Center ever talked to a class that you were in? _____ Yes _____ No

73. Did you ever go to see any of the Self Center staff while you were *in school?* _____ Yes _____ No

74. Think about all the visits you made to them *in school:* PLEASE CHECK *ALL THE REASONS YOU WENT TO SEE THEM IN SCHOOL:*

_____ To make a clinic appointment

_____ To talk about being pregnant

_____ To talk about V.D.

_____ To talk about birth control

_____ To talk about a problem

_____ For a movie or rap group

_____ Other: What? _____

75. Whatever method of birth control you are using, where did you get it the *last* time?

_____ Not using any method of birth control

_____ Self Center

_____ A friend or relative

_____ Another clinic

_____ A private doctor

_____ A drugstore

_____ Other: Where? _____

What method are you using now? _____

76. What best describes you and the Self Center on Caroline Street:

_____ I've never been there

_____ I've been there once or twice

_____ I've been there three or more times

When was the *first* time you went to the Self Center? _____ _____
MONTH YEAR

If you have *never been to the Self Center* go to Question #80. If you have been to the Self Center answer all of the remaining questions.

77. *If you have been to the Self Center,* which of these apply to you? (CHECK *ALL* THAT APPLY.)

_____ I got a contraceptive method at the Self Center (pill, diaphragm, foam, condoms). *Circle* which method(s) you got the *first* time you got a method from the Self Center.

Was that your first visit to the Self Center? _____ Yes _____ No

_____ I went for a pregnancy test at the Self Center.

_____ I went to the Self Center for medical problems.

_____ I saw a movie or film strip at the Self Center.

_____ I went to the Self Center to be with a friend.

*78. During the *year before* you first went to the Self Center did you get any contraception from a doctor or another clinic? _____ Yes _____ No
IF YES: What method did you get from the *other clinic or doctor* the *last* time you were there (*before* you went to the Self Center)?

_____ Pill

_____ IUD

_____ Diaphragm

_____ Condom

_____ Foam

_____ Other: What? _____

*79. Have you been to another family planning clinic or a doctor *to get a contraceptive method* since you first went to the Self Center?

_____ Yes _____ No

80. Check the *one* statement that applies to you about this year.

_____ The Self Center was my regular place to get contraception this year.

_____ Another Clinic (*not the Self Center*) was my regular place to get contraception this year.

_____ I got contraception from a private doctor this year.

_____ I only use a method of contraception I can get without going to a clinic or doctor.

_____ I don't use contraception.

_____ I don't have sex.

81. If you use the *Self Center, another* clinic or a *doctor for contraception* (*not a drug store*), please check *all* the reasons you use the place you checked in the previous question.

_____ (A) It's close to where I live.

_____ (B) It's close to where I go to school

_____ (C) It's the only clinic I know about.

_____ (D) It's *not* in my neighborhood.

_____ (E) It has the best hours for me.

_____ (F) It's the cheapest I know about.

_____ (G) The people there really care about teens.

_____ (H) The people there don't tell your parents you came.

_____ (I) My friends go there.

_____ (J) My (mother/doctor/other adult) chose it for me (CIRCLE ONE).

_____ (K) I went there for some other reason and decided to get contraception too.

_____ (L) If you have an important reason for using the place you use which is not listed above PLEASE WRITE DOWN YOUR REASON IN THIS SPACE.

_____

_____

NOW, WRITE THE LETTER OF YOUR MOST IMPORTANT REASON FOR USING THIS PLACE IN THIS BOX

[ ]

82. If you consider the Self Center your regular place to go for contraception, what would you do if there were no Self Center?

_____ Go to the clinic (or doctor) I went to for contraception before.

_____ Find another clinic (or doctor) for contraception.

_____ Use a method of contraception that doesn't need a clinic or doctor.

_____ Have sex without contraception.

_____ Not have sex.

83. If you *did not* consider the Self Center your regular place for contraception *this year*, CHECK ALL THE REASONS WHY.

_____ (A) I didn't need a clinic for contraception.

_____ (B) My family or friends go to another clinic.

_____ (C) I wanted to go on with a clinic I'd been to before.

_____ (D) I heard the Self Center might be closing.

_____ (E) I don't know about the Self Center clinic.

_____ (F) I don't know where the Self Center is.

_____ (G) I don't like the staff at the Self Center.

_____ (H) The Self Center is too close to home—I'm afraid my family will find out.

_____ (I) My parent(s) are against my going to the Self Center.

_____ (J) I don't want my friend(s) to know I go to a birth control clinic.

_____ (K) My friends told me the Self Center wasn't any good.

_____ (L) I thought the Self Center cost money.

_____ (M) The Self Center is too close to school.

_____ (N) The Self Center is too far away from where I live.

_____ (O) The Self Center doesn't have the kind of birth control I like.

What kind? _____

_____ (P) Other: What? _____

NOW, WRITE THE LETTER OF YOUR *MOST IMPORTANT REASON* FOR NOT USING THE SELF CENTER CLINIC AS YOUR REGULAR PLACE FOR CONTRACEPTION THIS YEAR.

84. To help you get to the Self Center, how important is it to have people from the Self Center *speak in your classrooms?*

_____ Very important—I wouldn't go to the Center without hearing them first

_____ Somewhat important—it helps

_____ I don't think it makes any difference

_____ Unimportant—it's a waste of their time

85. To help you get to the Self Center, how important is it to have people from the Self Center in school *for you to talk to?*

_____ Very important—I wouldn't go to the Center without talking to them first

_____ Somewhat important—it helps

_____ I don't think it makes any difference

_____ Unimportant—it's a waste of their time

86. Has the Self Center changed what you *feel* about getting pregnant while you're in school?

_____ Yes, a lot

_____ Yes, somewhat

_____ A little

_____ No, not at all

87. Has the Self Center changed what you *do* (or would do) to keep from getting pregnant if you have sex?

_____ Yes, a lot

_____ Yes, somewhat

_____ A little

_____ No, not at all

GO ON TO THE NEXT PAGE . . .

*IF YOU HAVE EVER HAD A BABY, PLEASE ANSWER THESE QUESTIONS (IF YOU HAVE HAD MORE THAN ONE BABY, PLEASE ANSWER THESE QUESTIONS ABOUT THE *LAST* BABY YOU HAD).

1. Does your baby live with you now? _____ Yes _____ No

   IF NO: Is the child

   _____ living with someone else in your family,

   _____ living with his/her father or father's family,

   _____ adopted

   _____ no longer alive?

2. Were you in school (or on vacation and planning to come back) when you got pregnant? _____ Yes _____ No

3. When you were pregnant did you leave school for a while or did you *stay* in school? CHECK ONE ONLY

   _____ I left school when I was _____ months pregnant (PUT IN NUMBER)

   _____ I went to _____ school(s) when
   (WRITE IN THE NAME OF THE SCHOOL(S))
   I was pregnant.

4. How soon did you go back to school after you had your baby? _____
   (If you had your baby during the summer vacation but started back to school in September, check here) _____

5. What is your relationship *now* with the baby's father (the partner you had when you got pregnant)?

   _____ We're married   _____ We go out once in a while

   _____ We're engaged   _____ We don't date but we're friends

   _____ We're going together   _____ We're not friends any more

6. Does the baby's father ever take care of the baby with you?

   _____ Yes _____ No

7. Does he ever take care of the baby when you are not there?

   _____ Yes _____ No

8. IF THE BABY IS LIVING WITH *YOU*, WHO USUALLY TAKES CARE OF YOUR CHILD: (Tell us who the person is, *not* their names. For example, MY MOTHER, MY SISTER, etc.)
   From morning until 3 in the afternoon?

   Schooldays _____

   Days when you are not in school _____
   From 3 in the afternoon until 8 at night?

   Schooldays _____

   Days when you are not in school _____

From 8 at night until morning?

Schooldays _____

Days when you are not in school _____

Do you think there will be any change in who takes care of your child next

year? _____ Yes _____ No

IF YES: What changes? _____

Why? _____

THANK YOU FOR YOUR HELP.

FEMALE VERSION (B)

Questions different from Female Version A—Questions 54–70

How many of these people are living with you at your house now? CHECK ALL THOSE LIVING AT YOUR HOUSE NOW.

_____ Mother (real)	_____ Stepmother	_____ Foster mother
_____ Father (real)	_____ Stepfather	_____ Foster father
_____ Grandmother	_____ Grandfather	

_____ Brothers (real, foster and step)   How many? _____

_____ Sisters (real, foster and step)   How many? _____

Others: _____

55. Did you ever have a sex education course in school?
_____ Yes _____ No

IF YES: Which school? _____
Did it tell you about:

A girl's coming on (her monthly period)	_____ Yes	_____ No
The risk of a girl getting pregnant	_____ Yes	_____ No
Being a teenage parent	_____ Yes	_____ No
Different kinds of birth control (contraception)	_____ Yes	_____ No
V.D. (venereal disease)	_____ Yes	_____ No

56. Have you ever talked with one of your parents about these things? with a friend? (IN EACH COLUMN CHECK AS MANY AS YOU WANT)

	Parent	Friend
A girl's coming on (her monthly period)		
The risk of a girl getting pregnant		
Being a teenage parent		
Different kinds of birth control (contraception)		
V.D. (venereal disease)		

57. When in the month is a girl most likely to get pregnant? (CHECK *ONLY ONE*).

_____ Right before her period begins (Right before she comes on)

_____ During her period

_____ Right after her period

_____ About two weeks after her period begins

_____ Anytime during the month

_____ Don't know

Are you sure? _____ or was that a guess? _____

58. What time do you have to be home at night?

Weekdays — 5 — 6 — 7 — 8 — 9 — 10 — 11 — 12 — no limit

Weekends — 5 — 6 — 7 — 8 — 9 — 10 — 11 — 12 — no limit

59. Does any adult in your home work regularly for pay?
_____ Yes _____ No

Is your family on Medical Assistance now? _____ Yes _____ No
Does anyone in your household get a Social Service check now?

_____ Yes _____ No

Does your family get food stamps now? _____ Yes _____ No
Does anyone in your household get an unemployment check now?

_____ Yes _____ No

PLEASE ANSWER IF THESE ARE TRUE OR FALSE FOR *YOU*:

	TRUE	FALSE
*60. My boyfriend would think I was too eager for sex if I was ready with birth control.	_____	_____
61. My boyfriend would understand if I said "no" to sex until we had some kind of birth control.	_____	_____
62. Birth control costs too much.	_____	_____
*63. I'm afraid to be examined so it would be hard for me to go to a doctor or clinic for birth control	_____	_____
64. I would be embarassed to buy any kind of birth control in a store.	_____	_____
65. I would only have sex if one of us was using some kind of birth control.	_____	_____
66. I would *not* want my parents to know if I were having sex with my boyfriend.	_____	_____
67. I would like to have a baby while I am in High School.	_____	_____
68. It is hard to talk to my boyfriend about using birth control.	_____	_____
69. It is easy to talk to my parents about sex.	_____	_____
70. Sex (going all the way) before you are married is wrong.	_____	_____
71. It's important to be married before you have a baby.	_____	_____

72. What is the highest grade in school or year of college *your mother* has completed? (CIRCLE *ONLY ONE*.)

Before High School   1 2 3 4 5 6 7 8 9

In High School   10 11 12

In College   1 2 3 4

More school *after* completing college   5

73. You need your parents' permission to go to a birth control clinic.

_____ True _____ False

74. A young person of any age can buy contraceptive foam, cream or condoms at a drug store without parents' permission. _____ True _____ False

75. Young people can get treatment for V.D. without parent's permission.

_____ True _____ False

76. A girl who wants to have an abortion can do it without telling her family

_____ Yes _____ No _____ Don't Know

77. Have you taken this Questionnaire before? _____ Yes _____ No

IF YES: How many times before this one?

_____ one time _____ two times _____ three times

beliefs

to pg. 150

MALE VERSION

The questions below are ones that are omitted or very different from the female version.

28. Have you ever been to a store to get condoms (rubbers)?

_____ Yes _____ No

Have you ever gotten them from a coin machine? _____ Yes _____ No
Have you ever gotten them from somewhere else?

_____ Yes _____ No
IF YES: When was the *first* time you got condoms
(rubbers)? _____ _____
MONTH YEAR

If you do not remember the month, was it:

_____ Winter (January/February/March)

_____ Spring (April/May/June)

_____ Summer (July/August/September)   in _____
YEAR

_____ Fall (October/November/December)

How old were you? _____ years old

29. Have you ever been to a birth control clinic? _____ Yes _____ No
IF YES: Did you ever go there with your girlfriend?

_____ Yes _____ No
The *first* time you went, was it the:

_____ Self Center

_____ Another birth control clinic

30. Have you ever come (for example, had a wet dream)?
_____ Yes _____ No
IF YES: How old were you the first time you came? _____ years old
When was this? _____ _____
MONTH YEAR

If you do not remember the month, was it:

_____ Winter (January/February/March)

_____ Spring (April/May/June)

_____ Summer (July/August/September)   in _____
YEAR

_____ Fall (October/November/December)

35. How old is your father? _____ years old

    How old is your father's *oldest* child? _____ years old

    Does your father live in your house now? _____ Yes _____ No
    How often do you see him?

    _____ Every day or so

    _____ At least once a week

    _____ At least once a month

    _____ At least once a year

    _____ Never

    I would be more likely to talk over a personal problem with:

    _____ My Mother

    _____ My Father

    _____ Neither

    _____ Both

36. Have you had a job in the past year where you got paid?

    _____ Yes _____ No

    IF YES: How many hours per week do you work?

    (PUT NUMBER) _____ hours per week during the school year

    _____ hours per week, in the summer

44. Have you ever made a girl pregnant?

    Yes _____ Please go right on. *to next question*

    No _____ Go to Question #52 on the next page.

45. *IF YES:* How many times have you made a girl pregnant?

    _____
    NUMBER OF TIMES
    How did these pregnancies turn out?

    How many _____ babies?

    (GIVE A NUMBER) How many _____ abortions?

    How many _____ miscarriages?

    _____ Don't know *adoption*

46. How many different girls do you think you have made
    pregnant? _____
    NUMBER

47. When was the *last* time you made a girl pregnant? $\underline{\hspace{2cm}}$ $\underline{\hspace{1cm}}$
MONTH YEAR

What was the result? $\underline{\hspace{1cm}}$ she is still pregnant

$\underline{\hspace{1cm}}$ baby

$\underline{\hspace{1cm}}$ abortion

$\underline{\hspace{1cm}}$ adoption
$\underline{\hspace{1cm}}$ miscarriage

$\underline{\hspace{1cm}}$ don't know

48. I wanted to get a girl pregnant because no one thinks you're a man if you don't prove you can. $\underline{\hspace{1cm}}$ True $\underline{\hspace{1cm}}$ False

60. Rubbers (condoms) are too much of a hassle and get in the way. $\underline{\hspace{1cm}}$ True $\underline{\hspace{1cm}}$ False

63. *Any* kind of birth control gets in the way of sex, so I wouldn't want me or my girlfriend to use it. $\underline{\hspace{1cm}}$ True $\underline{\hspace{1cm}}$ False

79. During the *year before* you first went to the Self Center did you buy any condoms (rubbers)? $\underline{\hspace{1cm}}$ Yes $\underline{\hspace{1cm}}$ No

80. *Since* you first went to the Self Center have you *bought* any condoms (rubbers)?
$\underline{\hspace{1cm}}$ Yes $\underline{\hspace{1cm}}$ No

Appendix D
Details of the Data Cleaning Process

he cleaning process is a delicate and important task. It is during this
process that internal consistency is checked, a crucial measure of
the reliability of the data. There are several kinds of inconsistencies
which can be observed, and it is the educated scrutiny of the researcher
which leads to a series of critical decisions as to what a particular kind of
inconsistency means. In some cases, a discrepancy between two variables
that one believes should agree reflects an important finding in itself. For
example, discrepancies between two attitudes on similar subjects are very
common, and should not be treated as aberrations or unreliable responses.
Sometimes inconsistencies are the result of a simple error; in these cases,
after returning to the original document, the researchers may be able to clear
up a mistake without violating the reliability of the data. Finally, there will
be cases in which there is a true contradiction, which cannot be cleared up
with reference to the original document. In that case, one is unable to use
the two pieces of information in association. The description that follows
presents the methods by which we addressed some of these discrepancies
without violating the reliability of the data.

In the Hopkins project, the survey data were cleaned in five steps. Steps
one, two, and five are mandatory for any data set; steps three and four are
more specific and can be tailored to individual needs. The first step in cleaning survey data is to get a list of the coded values for each variable. This is
most easily done with a frequencies procedure that is found in many computer statistical packages. These lists are examined for out-of-range values
and easy-to-spot inconsistencies between variables. Once these values and
the cases to which they belong are identified, the original questionnaires
belonging to these cases are examined to determine what the correct codes
should be. In the Hopkins project, this step included examining those forms
with a poor "quality value." If these forms were not usable, they were de-

leted from the file and counted as refusals. All changes based on this first step are made on the computer and the affected cases should be rechecked.

The second step in cleaning is to run crosstabulations; again, programs are available to do so. The purpose of this step is to compare items that are dependent on one another or in which the responses should have been consistent. Again, problems and cases are identified and examined, and changes are made and checked. One recurrent problem found in the responses to the Hopkins survey, by examining crosstabulations, was that students who checked "no" to a behavioral question, or who failed to answer it, would proceed to give subsequent information relating their experience with that event. For example, after indicating that they had never used contraception, they would check methods they had used. For each set of questions, we established rules by which we could consider the answer to the initial part to be affirmative. We retained codes to identify these cases, but with enough supportive evidence, felt free to consider that the respondents had, indeed, experienced the behavior.

The next two stages in data cleaning are more specific to the Hopkins project because of the nature of the information collected. However, they can be applied to any survey that asks for the recall of complicated information, such as dates and ages of events in complex histories. In the Hopkins project, the third stage of cleaning was a comparison of ages and dates of events, since both were asked. When asking for the date of an event, we asked for both month and year. Respondents were often given a list of seasons, with the months following in parentheses, and were told to check the *season* if they did not remember the *month*. In that case, the middle month of the group assigned to the season was used. If there was a discrepancy between the age and the date of the event the respondent gave, the general rule was to use the age and month that had been given, and to change the year to match. We believed that the recalled age would be closer to the truth than the month and year in which the event occurred, especially for events relatively far in the past. An exception was made for current age and date of birth. When they did not match, it was usually because a birthday was approaching, or had just passed, and the respondent had put the new or old age, respectively. In that case, the age was changed to match the date of birth. Similar adjustments were made for errors in age and date of last intercourse if the events were not too distant in time. Thus, very specific rules, based on our understanding of the original questionnaire, were consistently applied.

The next step in data cleaning was specific for the pregnancy information, as it was too important and too complicated to trust to the cleaning process previously described. Each questionnaire in which the respondent reported a pregnancy (or that he had made a girl pregnant) was examined individually. Consistency within the pregnancy information was checked as well as consistency between the pregnancy data and information about sexual intercourse. Variables were created by hand for the ninth- through twelfth-grade females to express whether or not they had ever been pregnant, and if so, how often.

At the end of the cleaning process, frequencies and tables were rerun to make sure there were no remaining data problems that still required attention.

Data cleaning can be tedious and unexciting. However, the more one does at this stage and the more rigid the rules that are enforced, the easier the data will be to use for analysis, and the more quickly the results will emerge. It is well worth the effort to create a clean, usable data set so that problems are not encountered later, perhaps when it is too late to do anything about them.

Index

About the Authors

Laurie Schwab Zabin is Associate Professor of Population Dynamics in the Johns Hopkins School of Hygiene and Public Health, with a joint appointment in the School of Medicine's Department of Obstetrics and Gynecology. She received her B.A. from Vassar College, her M.A. from the Harvard Graduate School of Arts and Sciences, and her Ph.D. in Population Dynamics from the Johns Hopkins University. Her career in family planning has included roles as provider, consultant, community organizer, and administrator, locally, nationally, and internationally. She served as Director of a Community Action Family Planning Center in Baltimore for the Office of Economic Opportunity and the Planned Parenthood Association of Maryland; she has also served as President of the Board of that association and received its Margaret Sanger Award. She has been on the Board and Executive Committee of the Planned Parenthood Federation of America, and recently served as Chair of the Board of Directors of the Alan Guttmacher Institute. She is on the Governing Council of the American Public Health Association representing the Population and Family Planning Section, of which she has served as chair. Her recent work has focused on issues related to adolescent pregnancy in the United States.

Marilyn B. Hirsch is an Assistant Professor in the Department of Gynecology and Obstetrics, School of Medicine, Johns Hopkins University, with a joint appointment in the Department of Population Dynamics, School of Hygiene and Public Health. She received a B.S. in biology and mathematics from William Smith College and a Ph.D. in population studies from Johns Hopkins University. She has worked at the Centers for Disease Control and at the National Center for Health Statistics. She played an important role in carrying out the 1979 National Survey of Young Women and Young Men, which was based at Johns Hopkins University. Besides the present work on evaluation, she has done research on contraceptive use, abortion, and infertility in the United States. She has also been involved in the areas of survey methodology, questionnaire construction, and data management. Dr. Hirsch received the Johns Hopkins University Alumni Association Award in 1980 and, in 1986, an award for the outstanding student/fellow research article published in the *Journal of Adolescent Health Care*. She is on the Board of Directors of the Maryland Women's Health Coalition.